Kundalini Yoga
Sadhana Guidelines
Create Your Daily Spiritual Practice
2nd Edition

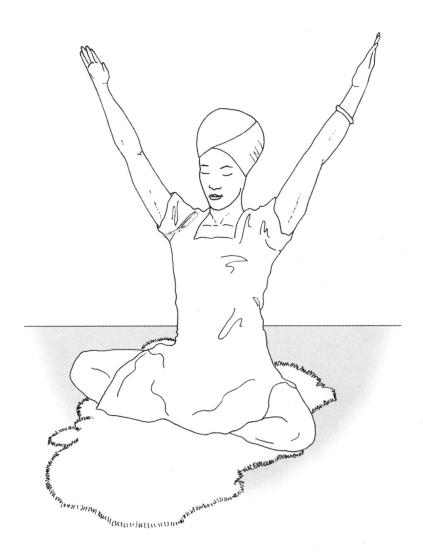

Kundalini Yoga as taught by Yogi Bhajan®

Kundalini Research Institute

ISBN 978-0-9786989-8-0
Managing Editor
Sat Purkh Kaur Khalsa

Senior Editor
Gurucharan Singh Khalsa, Ph.D.
Director of Training

Contributing Editor & Illustrator
Harijot Kaur Khalsa

Book Design & Production
Ravitej Singh Khalsa CVO
Tara Kemp (& Musical Notation)
Khalsa Marketing Group Inc.

Producer & Publisher
Kundalini Research Institute

FSC
www.fsc.org
MIX
Paper from
responsible sources
FSC® C008955

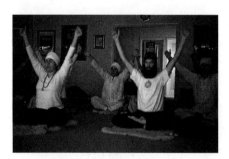

Rise Up, Rise Up
Sweet family dear
The time of Lord and remembering
Love is near
Love, love is all you say
If you'll awake and rise up
right away, hey hey
If you'll awake and rise up, right away

The Lord will bless you
In so many ways
If you will rise up right now
Sing His praise

Rise up, rise up sweet family dear
The time of Lord and remembering
Love is near
Love, love is all you say
If you'll awake and rise up
right away, hey hey
If you'll awake and rise up, right away

Guru Singh Khalsa

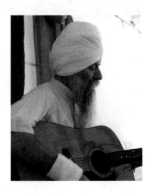

Acknowledgments

Kundalini Yoga Sadhana Guidelines would never have been possible without our teacher, Yogi Bhajan. From cover to cover, these are his teachings and our gratitude to him is infinite. I would like to acknowledge personally the input and advice given by Kundalini Yoga instructors across the country who have used the First Edition for their classes these past 30 years. It is through their dedication and service that we've been able to update this timeless manual.

In addition, we would like to thank the tireless efforts of Harijot Kaur Khalsa, who's dedication to the teachings has given birth to dozens of priceless yoga manuals over the years and the drawings in this book; and to the work of Ravitej Singh Khalsa, who created the original manual by hand more than 30 years ago and is still serving the teachings today in designing and delivering this Second Edition.

Gurucharan Singh Khalsa, Ph.D.

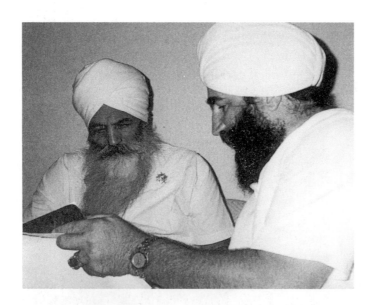

This manual is dedicated to Yogi Bhajan and to the Golden Chain of teachers and students extending from the Infinite to the One within, linking us all together through time and space as we are each, in turn, students to our teachers and teachers to our students.

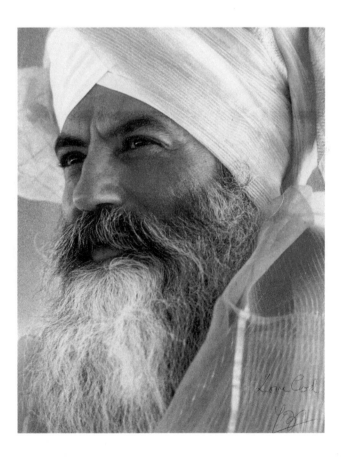

Hukam (Command)

Say, what lies with a man to do or not?

Only the Lord causes to happen what He will.

If man had the power, he would seize everything to himself.

But he can do only what the Lord wants done.

Not knowing this, man dwells with illusion,

For if he knew, would he not save himself?

But deluded by doubt, he wanders in all directions,

And rushes forth to explore all the four continents.

When, however, out of His Mercy, God grants His love,

Man absorbs himself in the practice of the Name.

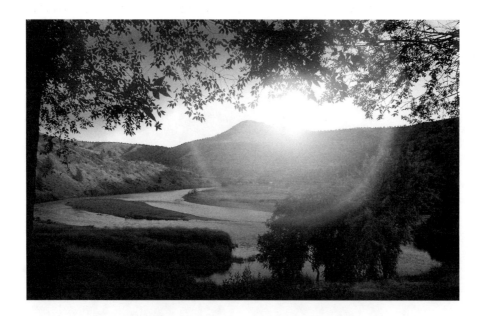

Foreword to the Second Edition

Originally a volume of the Kundalini Quarterly, *Kundalini Yoga Sadhana Guidelines* is a revision of the still older *Guidelines for a Successful Sadhana*, Volumes 4 & 5, of the *KRI Journal of Science of Consciousness for Living in the Aquarian Age*, published in 1974. Both the original work and this newest edition were compiled by Gurucharan Singh Khalsa, Ph.D.

This new edition includes an updated essay on Morning Sadhana from Gurucharan Singh, outlining many of the essential points from his original essay plus a review of all the sadhanas given to the 3HO community over the years and a perspective on the Aquarian Sadhana as it is to be practiced through the year 2012. The original essays from Yogi Bhajan on yoga and meditation can still be found plus a wealth of kriyas and meditations that you have come to know and love and a few new ones, favorites like Kriya for Morning Sadhana and Trishula Kriya.

This also marks a new beginning in our effort to serve the entire international community of trainers, teachers, and students. We will be publishing *Kundalini Yoga Sadhana Guidelines*, 2nd Edition, in two languages simultaneously, with further translations available in the months and years to come. We hope you enjoy this new edition and that with it you can approach this coming Age with gladness in your heart, steel in your veins, caliber in your character, and awareness in your consciousness to serve and uplift everyone you meet—just by your presence.

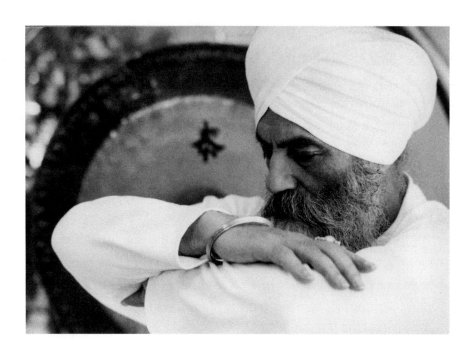

"Sadhana gives one a disciplined practice to integrate the body, mind and spirit."

–Yogi Bhajan

Contents

Kriyas

Meditations

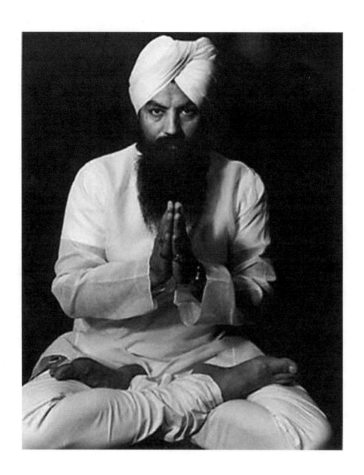

*Sadhana is self-enrichment. It is not something
which is done to please somebody or to gain something.
Sadhana is a personal process in which you bring out
your personal best.*

–Yogi Bhajan

Sat Nam! In January of 1969, when Yogi Bhajan first started teaching Kundalini Yoga in Los Angeles, California, I took notes. In longhand (sprinkled with a little shorthand), I wrote as fast as I could, because I knew the minute I walked out of the class, I wouldn't remember the timing, or even the sequence of the exercises, much less all the things he said that opened up a whole new world of awareness. He explained so much before, during, and after the exercises. He repeated many of the basic concepts over and over, and slowly we learned a new vocabulary. We learned new mantras. We began to experience the energy and the transformation that comes with the practice of Kundalini Yoga.

I used my notes when I began teaching in February of 1969. Soon someone was smart enough to start recording his classes. (It was probably Siri Ved Singh, to whom we owe a huge debt of gratitude, especially for capturing Yogi Bhajan's priceless lectures later on video! These early days meant using the big reel–to–reel tapes.)

But Yogiji wouldn't let us put anything in print for more than three years! He said it was important for students to study with a living Teacher. He wanted to ensure that people would not misinterpret the written words. He obviously knew how difficult it would be to learn from a book. It takes a lot of skill to present this sacred information clearly and in a form that avoids misunderstanding.

Finally, in 1972, he said okay. And I sat on my living room floor sharing all my notes and the notes taken by the first students like Mark Lamm, Guru Singh and Gurucharan. Gurucharan Singh Khalsa started the Kundalini Research Institute with Yogi Bhajan and compiled from all these notes the first edition of *Sadhana*

Guidelines as one of their first publications. That first edition was published in multiple languages with more than 100,000 copies bought and used worldwide. As the years passed, we realized the information and explanations needed more clarification and in some places correcting, so it is with great pleasure that we are now able to offer this expanded and improved edition (new illustrations, too!) of what I consider one of the most important and essential tools for any student or teacher of Kundalini Yoga.

I am grateful to have had a small part in the creation of this excellent publication. With deepest appreciation to Gurucharan Singh Khalsa, KRI Director of Training, and the entire staff of the Kundalini Research Institute, I'm proud to announce the second edition of *Kundalini Yoga Sadhana Guidelines*.

Humbly yours,

Shakti Parwha Kaur Khalsa
Mother of 3HO

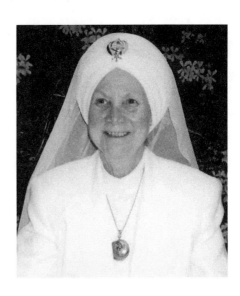

Introduction to the Second Edition

By Gurucharan Singh Khalsa, Ph.D.

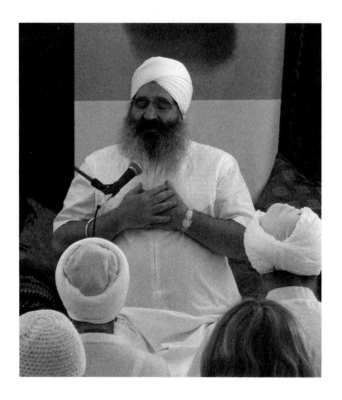

It is fascinating to look at what I wrote at the beginning of Yogi Bhajan's mission to teach, uplift and create a legacy of teachers for the future—and to now update it after 35 years. Yogi Bhajan was a precious fountain of teaching. He repeated key themes and elaborated on them with new techniques, delivered in a way that served the needs of his immediate audience as well as the potential of all those who would practice in the future. The basics of sadhana are perennial and remain the same. Over the years, after the first edition, he gave many different ways to practice morning sadhana. We include in this edition all of those practices along with a brief commentary on the purpose for each of them. Having this history of sadhana is important because his instructions for the future, as we leave the Piscean Age behind in 2011, include practicing all that he taught.

He worked relentlessly to give us the standards of a human being, the virtues we are capable of expressing, the character we can live by to be happy, and the practical tools we can use in Kundalini Yoga and Meditation to achieve them. He was practical, intuitive, and compassionate and challenged each of us to be happy, to be real and to share with every other human being the tools that he shared. His teachings and the sadhana practice he gave are authentic and embody the best of all the ancient traditions delivered and explained through the sensitivity of a Master. Each kriya and meditation is woven tightly into a perfect composition that is well tested and perfectly given—as a Beethoven would present a perfect combination of notes and harmonies that maximized the musical instruments and awakened the musical potential in each listener and player.

The future that we all face promises great challenge, great opportunity and great awakening. Competition will be global and intense, so we need the capacity and the power of a lifestyle that arises from spontaneous discipline. We need stillness in the midst of the blinding speed of change. We need depth to know our direction in life. We need caliber to deliver who we really are with elegant effectiveness. And we need unlimited compassion to understand each other in a world that knows no distance or privacy.

In other words we each need a sadhana. Sadhana may not produce a miracle for you, but it will give you the foundation and the energy to let the miracle of you shine forth! This new edition is here to serve you and to help you uplift yourself and others. The entire team of KRI and our global community of teachers are with you every morning, no matter where you reside, with prayers, blessings and gratitude.

This edition is needed to respond to a vastly increased community of yoga practitioners and to recognize the ongoing need for a focused, simple manual to help each person develop a personal practice of sadhana. The new edition efforts were spearheaded by Nirvair Singh Khalsa, brought to fruition with editing and production by Sat Purkh Kaur Khalsa, enhanced and updated by myself, illustrated by Harijot Kaur Khalsa, nurtured by Nam Kaur Khalsa and creatively assembled by Ravi Tej Singh Khalsa who was a great advocate of the value of this new edition.

Grateful in Service,

Gurucharan Singh Khalsa, Ph.D.
KRI Director of Training
May 14, 2007

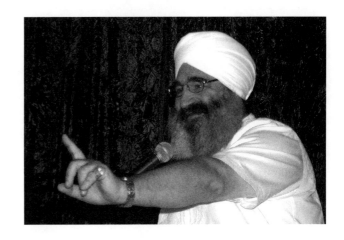

Introduction to the First Edition

By Gurucharan Singh Khalsa, Ph.D.

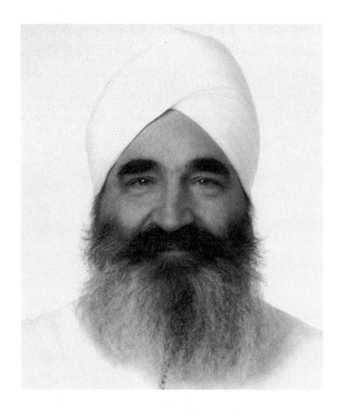

This manual is designed for both the new and the experienced student. It focuses on the essential practice of Kundalini Yoga—sadhana. Quite a bit of new material has been added since it appeared in KRI's *Journal of Science of Consciousness for Living in the Aquarian Age*. A section on basics and several beginner's sets are to aid the use of this manual in the many college courses now being taught. The three lectures by Yogi Bhajan were added to give a broader introduction to the nature of Kundalini Yoga and meditation.

All of the thought, inspiration, and techniques for this manual have come to us from Yogi Bhajan. His openness and true humility in sharing the knowledge and secrets of the sages, the truths distilled from ages

of human experience, is the keynote of the Aquarian Age. Any mistakes are those of this scribe, not of the teacher.

Yogi Bhajan spoke about sadhana at the Winter Solstice celebration in December, 1973, in Orlando, Florida. This excerpt from his informal talk summarizes the essence and spirit of all the pages to follow. If this statement is taken to heart and put into practice, all other questions will be answered.

"A *sadhu* is a being who has disciplined himself. Sadhana is the technique to discipline yourself. Those who create separation in sadhana have not yet crossed the barriers of their mind and ego. I will show you by example. I don't know how you can be so idiotic to say someone who is doing a sadhana can create terrible problems when actually he is blessed.

"Once we invited a teacher to Guru Ram Das Ashram and he chose to speak on Kundalini Yoga. He told me to come and sit by his side. I said, 'Nothing doing. You are my guest and at any one time, one teacher speaks.' So I made him sit there and I sat in the area where the students sit. We listened to 45 minutes of his speech against Kundalini Yoga, very calmly and very quietly, and it didn't bother us. In the end he asked me to give a closing remark. I got up and said, 'God bless you. You have given us a chance to know how faithful we are.' And that's it.

"A sadhana is a sadhana. In sadhana, if *Japji* is read, let everybody read it. Let everybody sing with it, let everybody glorify himself. Or if there is a Grace of God course, where the ladies are participating and they just want to participate separately, let the men go into silent prayer. Say, 'God, really make them a grace of God so that they will get off our backs!' Do you see what I mean? We can always help each other so that there is no problem. But we have a habit of doubting everything to the extent that we become a living doubt! Doubt, doubt, doubt, everything doubt.

"I feel that in the morning, when you go for sadhana, you are going to be sadhus. What does it matter if somebody just gets up to say, 'Hmmm Hmmm?' That person is still doing it! He is doing something; he is not sleeping. It is far better than a person who is snoring. Do you understand? Sadhana is a willful effort to prove you are not lazy about your own infinity. When the sun rises early in the day, even idiots rise; but blessed are those who rise before the sun to prove that they are sons of the Almighty. Does it sound clear to you? At 3:30p.m. you will probably get up. But those who have the guts will open up the gates of the heart at 3:30a.m., they will love their Lord, they will communicate with their God and they will tell him, 'Whether you belong to us or not, we belong to you.' That is all it's about.

"It is a time and a process where people get up in the morning to chant the glory of the Lord, in this way or in that way, and then they clean their temple. This is how sadhana takes place at the Golden Temple in Amritsar, India. When we first go to the temple, we take away everything, clean the floors, then give the marble a bath with milk. We clean and polish every part of it, then redecorate it. Then at 3:00a.m. the gates open and the sangat is allowed to come. The sangat chants there from 3:00 to 5:00a.m. and then, in a golden palki sahib, the Guru Granth Sahib is brought in. At 7:00a.m. the hukam [1] is taken. Those who have gone to the Golden Temple know it.

"In your own sadhana it is exactly the same way. Your body is the temple of God, and your soul is the divine Guru within. So you get up in the morning; you meditate; you chant the mantras; you do the exercises; you call on your spirit; you regulate the breath; and you get together in group consciousness because it helps each other. That is what morning sadhana and group consciousness is: It is a help to each other.

"If I am trying to sleep, another is not sleeping. If in this whole group one person opens up to God just once, we all will be blessed in his openness. That is what matters. If one has walked into sadhana with heart and soul in a prayerful mind, we will all be benefited. That is the power of the group sadhana. All should participate. But you know, we still have something of the past in us. We bring up worries about who should lead: 'Oh, that leader has brought a very good sadhana; that one has freaked out the sadhana.' We go through this every day. The truth is that nobody freaks out the sadhana and nobody makes it beautiful; it is the will of God which prevails through the soul. When you are a servant and act as a channel, it prevails through you; when you are clogged up and mugged up it doesn't come through. That's what it is.

"If in the morning sadhana there is somebody other than a Sikh (Sikh means a seeker of the truth), what can I say to him? If in the morning sadhana one cannot curtail the barriers and get to the oneness, I don't think there is any other time it can happen. One for all, because all is for one. That's the principle."

1. The Sikh scripture contains teachings and songs of divine inspiration of both Sikh Gurus and Hindu and Muslim saints and bards ranging from the 12th through the 17th centuries. A hukam is a verse chosen at random from the Siri Guru Granth Sahib, read each morning to the congregation as the direction for the day.

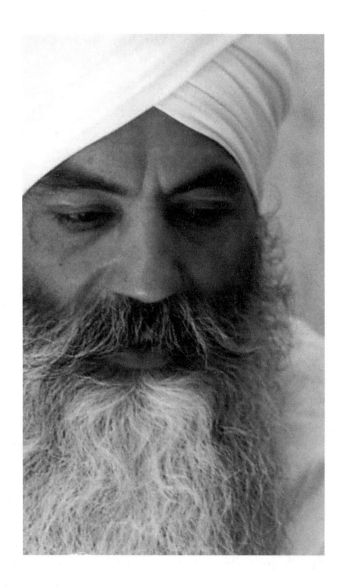

You can have a
healthy, happy, holy,
wholesome life,
a fulfilled life,
a beautiful life
in which you can
perceive in yourself
the contentment
of existence.

—Yogi Bhajan

An Adventure in Awareness
by Yogi Bhajan, Ph.D.

. . . People do not have a basic understanding about yoga. Some people think yoga is a religion. Some people think it is for vitality and health. Some people think it is to promote their personality. In reality, this is all a misunderstanding. The word yoga, as we in the West understand it, has come down from the biblical word, yoke. If you go to the original word in Sanskrit, it is *jugit*. The definition of a yogi is a person who has totally leaned on the supreme consciousness, which is God. Yoga is the union of the individual's unit consciousness with the infinite consciousness. That is all it means.

Classically, your potential self is infinite, whether you know it or you don't know it. The fact remains that every human mind belongs to infinity and to creativity. But in practical action, it is limited. So the technical know-how is required through which a man can expand his mental faculties in order to bring about the equilibrium to control his physical structure and experience his infinite self. That's all yoga means in very simple terms.

In this life of ours, yoga is greatly needed. Today the human being does not understand why he is a human being or what it means to be a human being. Talking about his infinity and knowing and experiencing infinity is a big deal. Remember that wisdom does not hold you. Wisdom only becomes knowledge when you experience it. Only the experience of that knowledge, *gyan*, can hold and support you. Just because you know or believe something to be true does not mean that you can act on it. But if you know truth and act on that path, and if you find bliss, success and fulfillment

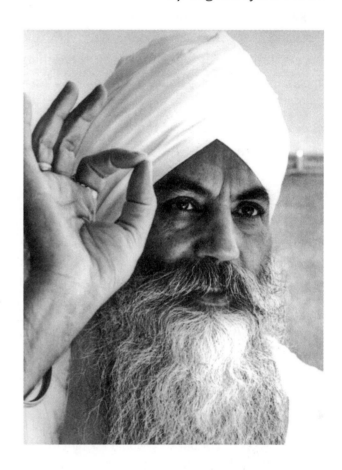

in yourself, then no power on earth can make you do wrong. Once you have seen the joy of that truth and have enjoyed that beauty you are okay. Some people misunderstand this. They say knowing the truth is alright. They say wisdom is good, but knowledge is not good. Wisdom becomes knowledge when it becomes your personal experience. And anything which can hold and support you is knowledge. A guru can give you wisdom but he cannot give you knowledge. And this is where we normally mess ourselves up. We think that so and so is a wise man. Learning from him, serving him, feeling good about him will make everything alright. But no, it never works that way. He can give you the technical know-how but the knowledge yours. His is the wisdom. So he has an essential part to play in this, but you are an equally essential part.

The first factor as a human being is to understand your vehicle, the physical or gross body. You have a very complicated inner machinery. It is not just the flesh and bones you can see. It's a very systematic system. It has glands, blood circulation, a breathing apparatus, heart-beat pulsation, a brain, and a total nervous system. All those systems combined over a structure of flesh and bone constitutes your physical system. It is a functional system. Whatever is a functional system needs cleaning, needs care, needs tuning. It also needs careful assessment of its capacity of activity, its potential to be extended, and its possibilities of longevity; all that has to be taken care of to start with.

If somebody wants to mess himself up all he has to do is overeat. After ten or fifteen days he'll be in the hospital. There's no problem. In New York I met a case. I said, "Why are you on welfare?" He said, "I can't hold myself together." It surprised me. His problem was that he overate. He would get sick and go to the hospital. After he got out they would ask him to take precautions and not do it again. But he would immediately overeat, get sick, and go back in. It was a chronic cycle.

The physical body is the basic temple in which you can deposit the treasure of happiness of life. You have to understand it. When you are young you can play mischief with the physical body. But in old age the body has you paying for the playing. You can never get out of it. So the body has to be scheduled. You have to calculate on a sliding scale. Suppose I must live a hundred years. Now, I have to plan for that. How should I carry this model 1929, or whatever model it is? From that year you want to live a hundred years. Now, if you buy a car in 1970 for a single driver, you

can expect that with regular service, oil changes, etc. that it will get a certain mileage. But if you do not schedule it practically, after two years you will have to buy a new car. You are very happy to change a car because it gives you status in society, and a new car is good to drive all the time. But it doesn't work that way with the human body. You are not so fearless that after five or ten years you can say, "Alright, I can change the human body, I can get into another." You have not developed your individual consciousness to universal consciousness so that you can do it. There are people, there have been human beings, who have done it. It's not an unusual feature. But mostly people do not know how to do that. Therefore it is essential to make the best of what you have.

In this course, we will study the human body in the light of yoga therapy to make it understandable to you and to show you how you can make the best use of it. You must be able to keep [your body] on the level of consciousness you choose, so that it can serve you better and better, without a lot of trouble. That's the maximum you can do.

A second factor in our human life is our mind. If the horizon of thought and understanding, tolerance and patience is limited, and if the mind is not so beautifully functional that it can see the unseen, and understand the consequences of actions, it is practically impossible to live a happy life; because if you do not have a road map, you do not know where you are going. Then what are you doing? Just driving? That's what we do in life. I don't want to pull your leg. I want you to feel very happy and good, but I have to give you a basic human assessment and overview.

What is the aim of your life? "Oh, everything is all right." What is all right? Nothing! Ask anybody. Everybody has twenty complaints about himself. Why? Where does the time go? Early in the morning, you go to the office and earn money. Saturday you have to pay your bills and buy the groceries. If there's a long weekend you have to take care of your taxes. Three hundred and sixty-five days go like this. Only leap year adds an extra day and that only comes after four years. We are that involved in life that we don't know any better. And when we do not know any better, how's the better going to come? We have passed our years with such speed that we do not know how we are maintained, except with God's blessing.

This functional structure of a human machine is so beautifully made by the Maker that it can recover from normal jerks and problems. It is a real and very rare mental shock that can damage your mental energy. When there is constant pressure and no relaxation, when there is no outlet, or when there is constant boredom in life, or a constant cavity in the capacity of mental life, it results in a shattered mind and the loss of happiness. Then you must get to a psychiatrist or a counselor or some yogi or do something. You have to depend on someone. Then every wise man will put a string in your nose and carry you through. But I don't believe in that. I believe every man represents God.

There are three basic letters in the word "God": G-O-D. These letters stand for the generating principle, the organizing principle, and the destroying principle. What we have done is taken the first letter from each of those three words and combined them together to make the word "God." God is not a guy standing on a seventh sky at the head of time watching you. It is the generating principle. It is infinity to infinity in relationship to the total creativity. Through its changing, everything happens. We have been brainwashed, but that has to be clearly understood.

We always say, "When I pray, God will come." What is prayer? Have you ever understood what a prayer is? You create a vibratory effect, it goes into the infinite creativity around your psyche, and the answer comes and is expressed in the energy of a job done. Then you say, "Well, prayer works." It is only your mind which has the power to concentrate and to work with that beauty.

Remember you have three aspects. You have the lower self, the gross or physical self; you have the central self, which is known as the existing self; and you have the higher self, which is a powerful, sophisticated and delicate self. So you can work on any level and you can go up and down, but you have to train yourself through your own experience. You can get knowledge from A, B, and C. It doesn't matter. If you can get wisdom from anybody, it is always a beautiful bounty. It is a special treat if you find some person who can stand by you and let you go through that experience. You are a God-conscious individual because you have the power of mental infinity.

I am talking in two languages now. In one word I am saying it scientifically, in the other I am relating in a mystic language. This way you can understand both. When you say, "I am a God-conscious person," it only means that you realize your mental capacity and ability. There is nothing more than that because everything you have is your mind. If somebody is beautiful or ugly to you, it is your mental evaluation. Somebody seems rich to you even though he doesn't give you a penny. He is rich to you because of your mental appraisal. You may imagine somebody is poor, even though the guy may have a million dollars sitting right under his seat. You call him poor because of your own mind. Actually, everything is your mental outlook. The problem with your mind is that as you think, so you are. How can man develop his mental faculty to perceive everything correctly? I would like to train you in that capacity so that you may have a happy life around you.

The third factor as a human being is the soul, the spirit. As no lamp can burn without methylated spirits in it, so no life can exist without a relationship of spirit in it. Spirit has many meanings, tones and facets. If there is a central thread in it, it is the general flow of the cosmic energy. In Catholicism we call it God; in yoga we call it cosmic energy. The meanings are exactly the same.

You have to understand your physical relationship with that infinite energy and how you can tune in for your own purposes; so that you can have a healthy, happy, holy, wholesome life, a fulfilled life, a beautiful life in which you can perceive in yourself the contentment of existence. You should be so contented that if you had to quit this planet you would just say, "Thank you." You have got to give thanks. And if the bad times are coming, just say, "Wonderful." Good days are coming, say, "Fine."

After all, what is life? It is a wave. The light must follow the night as night must follow the day. Sunshine must follow the clouds, clouds must follow the sunshine. But you feel you are really something special. You want sunshine all the time. If man is in the sun all the time the nose gets burned and the eyes can't see. No one can live in this world with sunshine all the time. Is there anyone willing to do that? No. This up and down is the beauty. Having happiness all the time is a very boring thing. You can't live that way. You have to have a little pull sometimes and just feel where you are and where you should be. That's why we call this life a vibration. What is a vibration, actually? Vibration is that which vibrates. And what is that? A path of vibration. Up and down! A wave. As a wave moves, so life moves. What do we want out of it? What do we desire? We desire a mind which is neutral, which understands the wave. You all know about surfing? When there are heavy tides people go surfing. They enjoy it. Other people go crazy. A mind which is developed, artistic, and self-controlled rides on those waves in life and enjoys it

If a person with such a mind experiences a bad time, he can sit down and say, "Oh, God! Wonderful! What do you want? A bad time? So, what's it to me? I don't care." He communicates, he talks, he feels the fun. He's not upset. He knows after this night there will be a good warm day. He's going to have a lot of fun. So he preserves his energy. He keeps himself together. When the time comes that he can expand and enjoy, he comes out with all his energy to enjoy it all the way. That quality of mind has to be developed; it has to be trained; it has to be made and felt. The faculty and the capacity of the mind must be geared into those grooves of action. If that is not possible, nothing is possible. This process is another important part of yoga.

Actually Kundalini Yoga means awareness. Awareness is a finite relationship with infinity. That's what it means. This dormant energy is in you. This awareness is sleeping in you and you only experience your capacity within a limit. But when it can be extended to infinity you remain you, anyway. But in that state there is nothing lacking. This is what is called the basic human structure, the framework through which we have to function. Do you like it? Are you willing to agree to all this? I'm going to focus on this structure and its work. I do not know whether you will agree with me, and I don't want you to agree with me. Remember one thing: don't agree with me anywhere. If you have any point of disagreement, come out with it. I love argument, but I want another man to provoke it. I don't want to put a question in the mind of the people.

We all want to have good health. Many people feel we get sick because we do not know better. My personal feeling is very different. I don't believe that anybody wants to be unhealthy. But I also don't believe that we do not go and get sick. We do. We go and get sick sometimes.

There are two types of sickness: intentional and unintentional. Intentional sickness is when we know we are going to get sick but we still do it. I get into intentional sickness very often and I know that. Do you think a man of my awareness is an idiot? For eighteen days I didn't get any sleep and I am not aware that I'm going to get into trouble? From the day I put myself on the plane and started on tour until I returned today I didn't get the chance to sleep even though I tried. The schedule was automatic, the demand was heavy; from one meeting to another meeting, discussion after discussion, etc. We opened up our drug program with a press conference in Washington. After that everybody became curious. The news spread. Then people would not let us sleep. The subconscious mind did not allow us not to do sadhana. We also let anybody who wanted to talk to me have a chance. If somebody wants to know something we must share with him. You sometimes ask why I just don't share. But I can't do that. I thought we would have five days of rest in Canada. To my surprise they had a full schedule and I said, "Alright. We will not go by any schedule. Anybody can come in." That was the only way to safeguard that all the services would be completed. I was aware that I was getting sick intentionally. The body can only go to a certain extent. You can ride a horse and you can go on beating it; but it can only go a certain number of miles before it will start dropping. These are intentional sicknesses.

There are also unintentional sicknesses. For that I have a lot of compassion. We do not know how to eat, we do not know how to digest, we do not know how to live, we do not know how to take care of this body, and we do not worry about whether our glands are functional or whether our nervous system is all right. We do not know to check if our cleaning is perfect or our rest and activity are balanced. That is unawareness. And that makes us sick. And that is where the main pain lies. This is especially true in this society today.

This morning I was talking on television. I told them that I had to catch a flight and I had to go. They said, "Well, you cannot leave that way. We definitely have to talk to you. Not all the people could come to that church to see you because the church had a limited space; it couldn't hold more than five hundred people. The people have forced us to have you come and answer certain questions on the television." I think TV is the best way to get into the living room without breaking into the house. Television is quite a procedure. You get into that box and you talk about anything you like.

When I went on that program they were having a discussion with a trained specialist, an expert, who does not believe in marriage. He feels marriage is going to be wiped out of the Western countries. It is the most unrequired thing of the past. I asked him, "Then why are you talking about it?" He said, "I don't think it's essential." I said, "Well, your mother must have married your father. That's why you are discussing it with me today. Your existence is out of that action which should come out of the matrimonial relationship." And he said to me, "I want to ask a question." I said, "Well, go ahead. You are very anti-marriage and I am very much for it. You are an outcome and a by-product of a marriage. Therefore, you cannot speak too heavily against it." We had twenty minutes of laughing and happiness. I enjoyed it and he enjoyed it. Later on when the interview was over he said, "I am a great fool. I have made a total idiot of myself before all of Canada. (This was a coast-to-coast program.) What have I done to myself? I thought you were a simple yogi and that I would take you left and right." I said, "I am very simple. That's why I asked you very simple questions. You thought that by asking me two or three of the intellectual type questions you could just blow me up. But that is not true. You have to raise your mind to the capacity of my mind, and you will overcome it. If you don't have that mind, you are limited. You are just intellectually trying to argue left and right. But what is left and right about truth?"

To approach yoga in its totality, you have to know what living is; you have to know what a relationship

...t values this life can give you. If you know you want then you can find it. Without any ...ledge, are you just going to close your eyes and start walking? Where will you go? "I am going to the beach." You don't know. You may end up in the mountains. You have to keep yourself aimed. Your compass must tell you at what altitude, latitude and longitude you are going. It is a totally planned life because the "O" in the word "God," G-O-D, means organization.

We often misunderstand or deny our basic nature in our social habits and communication. First of all, we are people of faith. Our first impulse and our greatest capacity is faith. Suppose we find a happy man. We know he is a good man and that he talks truthfully. We believe him. If he says something, we can act on it, and we can get happiness. Then we share it. But we do not relate this way. Instead of receptivity, we say, "Well, why are you happy? Convince me before I listen. I don't believe you." We always live on our insecurity. We cannot hide it. We cannot discuss anything with any other human being without first questioning his personality. "Who are you? What are you doing? How can you say that?" Why do we ask these questions? First of all, we do not know who we are.

Actually, we can go through life in two styles: We can act as if everybody were thieves until proven saints. Or we can act as if everybody were saints until proven thieves. Which style of life your mind has as a conception and as an action depends on how strong a nervous system you have. People who live one style walk in every walk of life with an even attitude. If you ask them, "How are you doing?" They reply, "Oh, I am fine." If there are certain dangers they might encounter they say, "Oh, I don't care. No danger is going to bite me." People who live in the other style are completely different. If you tell them, "The road is clear. It has been checked. It is beautiful;" they will say "Oh, I don't believe it. I can't go. I can't walk further."

The basic insecurity in mental attitude and structure is often very elemental to a person's consciousness. I counseled a particular case in Washington, D.C.; we discussed everything. There was a little marriage dispute, something normal. We cleaned it out. But then the man said, "I understand that she has understood the mistake and when she understands, she never acts wrongly. But still, I can't believe her." She said with anger and frustration, "The thing that bugs me the most is that he always says he can't believe me!" When I went deeper into his personality I found that his not believing the woman came from his background of experienced knowledge that he got from the activity of his mother. It took me four hours to tell him, "Your mother was your mother, and this woman is your wife." He said, "That is my problem. I can't always believe it." So I said, "What are you up to? Don't you understand that she is your wife, not your mother? Why do you want to punish this lady because of your mother?" Then he told me that he had spent thousands of dollars going from one expert to another and still didn't know anything better. I said, "Alright. I'll tell you another way. Go and buy beads." So he bought the beads the next day. I said, "When you talk to [your wife], catch your beads with a hand. Forget you are talking for a few seconds and remember that you are catching something." He said, "What does that do?" I said, "It will remind you that you are talking to your wife, not your mother. Simple. Whenever you talk to this lady who is your wife, put a hand on the beads and remember that you are not talking to your mother. You are talking to your wife. You married her. She's your life partner." He said, "Well, a woman is a woman." I said, "But with this woman you share a bed. With your mother you don't. You were a little child when you did that. So please be mature." I had to be practical and go very deep into his basic foundations of life in order to dig him out of his insecurity. Then he could start a new life by himself.

In every mental state of mind the subconscious plays a large role of which we are not aware. We all think we know "my past." There is no such thing as "my past." That past is only the experience you have in your subconscious mind and it does not let you move forward in your life. In Kundalini Yoga, we fry this subconscious mind. We make a toast out of it and eat it. It is one of the best dishes we make. We have the technical know-how to approach this subconscious mind which sits behind our mind and does the mischief. That is what subconscious mind is. It sits in the back and can spoil the image of human life by repeating experiences which have already been tasted and are recorded in the subconscious mind. So the subconscious mind must be taken care of and trained to be an aid to life.

Another pattern that must be confronted in Kundalini Yoga is our self-belittlement and the feeling that we are very limited. "Oh, I, a poor humble self, can't do this. I am very miserable." We can play this game. There are three ways of playing it. Sometimes we play it to get sympathy from people, sometimes we play it to get recognized, and sometimes we really play it and we actually feel it. Everybody does it. It's just a matter of degree. Someone does it one percent; another does it one hundred percent. It means your activity in realizing your mental capacity is just that limited. You have not realized that your mind has an infinite horizon. There's actually no end to it.

Understand this today: There are no two people who are alike. Neither are they physically alike, nor are they mentally alike. They have only one likeness: The input of infinity can be equalized to the output of infinity—and that is the only thing in us which counts. We can all reach the state of infinity, of bliss, of nirvana. There are two hundred words for it. You can call it anything, it doesn't matter. But that's what it is.

Now I'll touch on a controversial point. Whatever religion you follow, no matter what you call it, you follow something meant for you to know your origin, which is infinity. That religion should get rid of your self-belittlement and limitation and lift you to your full human capacity. Instead, what you usually end up knowing is prejudice; division of humanity; love and hatred on the basis of belonging to certain thoughts, or certain feelings, or certain practices. This has done more harm to humanity than the good the religions were intended to do. Today, we do not even understand the basic word "religion." It comes from *religio* and means looking back at your origin. And what is your origin? Spirit! And what is your end? Spirit! So what are you fighting about? What is the discussion? If you are constant and under all given circumstances you relate to one thing—that you are a part of Infinity and you always lean on that power—then you'll never be unhappy. It is a practice.

We have never trained our minds to know our origin which is Infinity. Instead we have run into rituals. All these churches, temples, and synagogues, all the places of worship were meant to create group consciousness. We start with consciousness then progress to group consciousness and universal consciousness. These religious places were designed so that all the people believing one way could come and join together to praise the Lord and feel high. That was the purpose. But now people come there to fight elections and to think who should control the synagogue or church. Or the minister speaks and lays his number. It has become a regular mechanized ritual—a systematic system within the system. The purpose which was to get together to practice and feel and experience the group consciousness is gone. Man has become confused. For when a person does not have individual consciousness and does not develop that individual consciousness to a group consciousness, he cannot attain the universal consciousness. Barriers shall exist. And these are those barriers which keep a man limited. The development of group consciousness in the experience of infinity is the bridge to universal consciousness and the release of the unlimited self.

All the technology you need is in Kundalini Yoga. But we have a mental sickness. We are not constant at anything. If you are very regular, if you practice so that you can cater to yourself and have a better experience, you will enjoy your life more and extend its length. Hopefully, you will do your best. This knowledge and exchange is a brotherhood; it is a mutual existence. There's no big and no small. It's a sharing. It's very much a sharing. So if you are willing to get into that kind of sharing, that kind of love, that kind of existence, you are welcome. Otherwise, we are happy, you are happy. Wherever you are, you are; wherever we are, we are. There's no problem.

Man exists to help those who need existence. I always feel that pushing knowledge on people is pushing drugs. Pushing is pushing anyway, so I don't want to be a pusher of anything. That is something which I have never done in my life. I'm not going to push heavy knowledge on you, but I'd like to share with you certain things so that we can experience certain things.

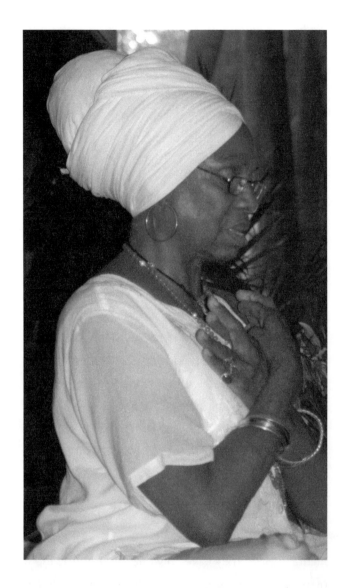

In Kundalini Yoga the most important thing is experience. Your experience goes right into your heart. No words can be said because your consciousness will not accept them. Your mind may or may not. All we want to do is to extend your consciousness so you may have a wider horizon of grace and of knowing the truth. Then you can smoothly plan your life to any extent you like. You can radiate creativity and infinity in all aspects of your daily life. Thank you very much. . . . God bless you.

Kundalini Yoga and Human Radiance

by Yogi Bhajan, Ph.D.

Tonight I would like you to ask any questions you like about Kundalini Yoga, its nature or history

Question: I have a friend who is a psychotherapist. He teaches Hatha Yoga as part of his therapy. He was telling me that Kundalini Yoga is an extremely dangerous form of yoga and can possibly lead to insanity if not handled right. Is this true?

Answer: It is very unfortunate that some people talk that way. First of all, they do not know what they are talking about. Second, they don't have any real experience of it. Actually, Kundalini Yoga produces whole human beings, teachers, and yogis. A yogi is one who has a union with the supreme consciousness. Some people teach it as if it is a bunch of dumb exercises, but they have no right to call themselves yogis. If flexibility in postures is the only yoga, then people in the circus are the best yogis.

Question: He doesn't consider himself a yogi. He just mentioned that he thought that Kundalini Yoga is a very dangerous aspect of yoga.

Answer: Ask him why he is practicing all the Hatha Yoga postures. What is the purpose of Hatha Yoga? The purpose of the Hatha Yoga is to raise the awareness. It is a technology to bring the apana and prana, the moon and sun powers, together to raise the consciousness through the central equilibrium line. In other words, its stated aim is to raise the kundalini. That is the purpose. But the problem is that it takes about 22 years to raise it that way, even with perfect

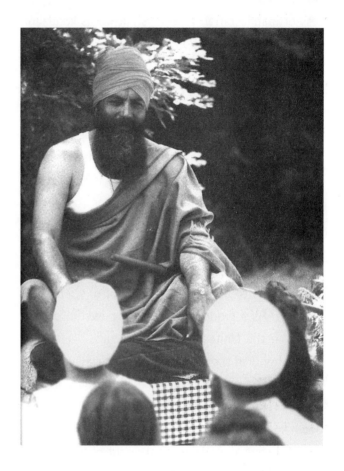

practice. That is the long method. It is a question of time only. Purpose is the same.

Teaching Hatha Yoga and Kundalini Yoga is very different. First of all, it is difficult to teach Kundalini Yoga. A man who does not have a beam of energy within himself cannot teach it. That is the first fundamental. You have to be aware in consciousness. It is a matter of a level of consciousness. You should be at a certain steady level of consciousness to pull all the people up to that level. That is the real problem. You could come and I could give you a bunch of exercises. You would feel good, but when you talk about life and humanity and the total sum of existence and consciousness, then you have to feel that magnetism come out of me. If I can't give you that, there is nothing to pull you to that level. That is the basic difference.

Let's talk this way. Actually, there was a God. He uncoiled himself, opened himself up. This uncoiling process or manifestation process is known as kundalini. What is dangerous about it? What is going to be uncoiled in you is already in you. It is an unlimited power and it is going to uncoil in you. There is danger when something outside is artificially put in you. But your system is already built to contain the energy of kundalini. You simply are not utilizing that energy. If you start utilizing that energy, where is the danger? This talk of danger sometimes becomes the biggest danger—and an even bigger problem. All these yogis love me but they do not feel very good with me. They love me because, as a Master of Kundalini Yoga, it is very difficult to hate me. It takes a lot of strength to hate me. As a group we are a very powerful organization in the United States of America. We have a couple hundred thousand people. Name a large town and there is a center nearby. The growth has all happened in three years. It is basically very difficult to put down somebody with that kind of following and that kind of personality. Where is the root of the distrust and warnings? Why is Kundalini Yoga put down? It is done either out of ignorance—or simply because I teach it! It has never been taught publicly before. The other yogis feel guarded about the knowledge out of a sense of national and racial loyalty. You understand that India was conquered by the British people who were Christians. So the lower classes and working classes of India were converted to Christianity. Traditionally, in India, this class of people is called untouchable. The majority of the Christians came from the untouchables, so even now in their minds and hearts a Christian is still untouchable. They feel this great sovereign secret of Kundalini Yoga was supposed to be learned only by highly special Brahmins. Now

this Yogi Bhajan got hold of it and he is just freaking out and giving it to every American without discrimination. It is very dangerous. It is dangerous culturally.

When I went back to India where I lived for 39 years, the one question everybody asked was, "What are you doing? What do you want to do in that country? Why are you teaching them?" All my friends were upset about it. They were not happy. When I told them Americans have the potential to experience the infinity, they said, "Oh, no, no, no. What has gone wrong with you?" When they started questioning me, I withdrew and said, "Alright, I am happy with my Guru, what do I care. It is my destiny."

There are certain things in my life which I can't overcome. They are in my destiny. I never came to this country by my own choice. I had no means to reach all these people who have come to know me. People have come to me. I have never even thought or intellectualized for a moment and said, "I did it." What I feel is that those souls who have to come and learn from me are already in the body. I already have this knowledge which I am to share with them, so all I end up being is a postman to deliver their letters. When my mailbag is empty I can quit. That is how I feel.

What is kundalini, actually? You experience it when the energy of the glandular system combines with the nervous system to create such a sensitivity that the totality of the brain receives signals and integrates them. Then a person understands the effect of the effect in a sequence of the causes. In other words, man becomes totally and wholly aware. We call it the yoga of awareness. Just as all rivers end up in the ocean, all yogas end up raising the kundalini in man. What is the kundalini? It is the creative potential of the man. In one year, about one hundred and thirty-five thousand people have practiced Kundalini Yoga and we have heard no complaints whatsoever.

Somebody may want to talk out of jealousy or ignorance, but we don't have to answer to that. What is God-consciousness? What is Christ-consciousness? What you call Christ-consciousness, we call kundalini. When man uncoils his potential—in activity—that is what it is. When I started teaching Kundalini Yoga everybody told me, "It will not be popular, you should start with Hatha Yoga." I am a good Hatha Yogi. When these Hatha Yogis get sick, I treat them. I have a specialty in yoga therapy, where you use Hatha Yoga postures and certain mudras and certain kriyas. But I chose not to teach just Hatha Yoga. When I came to this country, I had to decide, "Am I going to do it for myself or am I going to do it for these people?" I felt that the people here needed the type of system which could give them a positive result in realization in a very short time. There is no better system known to me than Kundalini Yoga. Raj Yoga is very mental and a student has to be very prepared for it. The beauty of Kundalini Yoga is that if you can just physically sit there with your pranayam automatically fixed, then with it, your mind is fixed. So a complete physical, mental and spiritual balance is achieved immediately, in one kriya. That's why it works so effectively in a short time.

To achieve universal consciousness through any method you have to raise your kundalini. To do this, a little technology and science is needed. After the eighth year of life, the pineal gland does not secrete fully. It needs to get the reserve energy that is stored at your belly button area, the navel point. That energy which developed you and gave you this shape and brought you on this earth has absolutely no residue. It is a pure energy. Do you understand what I am saying? That pure energy is still there. All you have to do is uncoil that energy and make a functional connection with your pineal gland. Once that master gland—the seat of the soul—has started secreting, it will give you the power to reach your self-realization in relationship

to the total universal awareness. Scientifically speaking, that is what must happen. But some people are still ignorant. If I had talked a hundred years ago about atomic energy people would have said, "Oh, it is dangerous. It is impossible. Who wants to do that?" First of all they didn't know about the atom. It is a human problem, not an individual problem. Without knowing anything about what something is or what something actually means, we only have opinions; and not only do we have opinions, we have set opinions!

Occasionally you will find an awareness which is unique in certain people who may not be practicing Kundalini Yoga but are known as having a sixth sense. They have inborn capacities. They have some intuitive power which tells them that the consequences of certain sequences of actions will be disastrous in the end. If you have this intuitive relationship between the individual consciousness and universal consciousness, you can compute what someone is trying to say before they say it. What they actually say is unimportant. You will know what they intend and what they mean. It is not very difficult. If a man comes to you, you may not even let him talk. You just say, "Well, you have come and you are ultimately going to ask me for a hundred dollars, but friend, I don't have it." I used to do that sometimes but people started sending word that I am a great psychic. That is not a good reputation so now I am very quiet about it. This intuitive capacity is natural. Actually, you become sensitive to the auric radiance of another person. As the signal comes, all you have to do is compute it and you will know what he is talking about. His words do not mean anything. You already know what he means. Most people are not aware that they have this ability in them. But with a little mental work, it can be achieved.

Our life as it is today has one basic human problem. We have to understand: A is A, B is B, C is C. Because

C doesn't understand what C is, he cannot understand what B is and what A is. And that is the total conflict in this world and it is a source of unhappiness to the human being. If C understands what C is, in that understanding his relationship with B and A will be very clear, and there will be no place for doubt. Because C doesn't understand what C is, C doesn't understand what B is either; but he wants to express himself about B and A. This kind of expression which is not based on a clear understanding will always be misguided. That is why this world has become a puzzle to us. Actually, the world is very clear. We are all human beings on this planet. We are supposed to live with each other in love, work as worship, and follow the path of righteousness, goading our lives through the time cycle of human energy to get across to infinity.

Why do we not fit in, in spite of the fact that we have the ability to fit in? There may be an ordinary man who is a grade B medical student. He gets a great opportunity. He rises above everything to the top. Then there may be a doctor who is a very brilliant student at college, but he never gets the opportunity. The confusion occurs when in spite of our equipped personality, we sometimes do not thrive and we do not understand why. There is a way to make sense out of this. We understand it intuitively, but scientifically it takes a little time.

According to the yogis, the symbol of man is the arc of life that we call an aura. The human aura is the arc of life. It is brilliant and white. Human existence depends on that arc. Most people can't see it and can't understand it. If you can see it, you can recognize the state of disease as well as the abilities of a person. All energy in existence has its own cycle just as this human being has his own cycle. That's what makes a human being unique. Every magnetic field has to cross this magnetic field of your arcline. The strength of the magnetic field of your arc determines how the other magnetic fields can or cannot enter and affect you.

Now a question arises. If there is a positive opportunity or vibration, will this arc of light reflect it so it won't enter? No! That positive energy will merge in it and will relate to the earth. If it is negative, it will be cancelled out at the arcline. Any person whose mental vibration results in a strong arc will protect all fragile areas of his life automatically with that arc.

When the magnetic field is strong, you relate to emotions differently. You can choose to relate to someone or disconnect from their influence. When your radiance is strong and you direct it to someone, they will want to talk to you and be around you in spite of great differences or pains. When man has the energy and he has the power through his psyche to relate or to forget, then he has nothing to worry about. The projection of his magnetic field will arrange the rays of his existence so that his psychoelectromagnetic circle can organize all the surrounding magnetic fields in tune with him. In other words, the environment will operate in tune with his purpose.

Let me say this in spiritual language. When the divine source that prevails through the man projects out the light of God, all darkness will go away. Wherever he shall go, there shall be light, beauty, bounty and fulfillment. These two explanations are the same, but one is in mystic language and the other is in scientific language. Kundalini Yoga is the science of changing and strengthening the radiance to give expanded life and capacity.

I'll give you an example of understanding human behavior with these two languages. Whenever the individual consciousness, while radiating, feels a cut or dip in the area of radiance, the connection that is trying to be made is not complete. When there is a cut, you cannot radiate correctly and the cycle of energy cannot complete itself into a creative action. What is a cut? A cut is division of energy.

Question: Well, what would cause a cut like this?

Answer: I am coming to that. We all have set patterns of behavior on which the pattern of consciousness is based. These patterns hold our personalities. A Hindu, for example, cannot eat meat because in his consciousness he feels it is a sin. A Muslim cannot eat pork because in his consciousness he feels it is a sin. A Christian eats meat and pork, because in his consciousness it is not a sin. Your consciousness must form a pattern of flow. Once you fix the pattern and frequency of that flow, then any time that your needs conflict with that established pattern, you cannot radiate. That's why some people cannot look into your eyes and talk, and others don't like to face you. What is wrong? Nothing, but a pattern of flow has been set. It is a combination of social environment and inner environment that forms the patterns. Those patterns form cavities in the aura. A cavity in consciousness is a duality. We act but we know that we don't think about it. Whenever your intellect, the giver of the thoughts, does not correspond to your set behavior, you have a problem.

In church, we would say that this is the conflict of a sinful man. What happens when you go and confess to a minister? What does he give you? Does he have some key to bind you up? No, you pour yourself out and he tells you that you are forgiven. You have a set pattern of belief in him; therefore, you can believe him and you can go on. Whenever something bothers you, there is only one way to get out of it. You have to have a captain, you have to have a person who will not betray your faith and who will counsel you to return to the path of righteousness. In other words, he should set the flow of the psyche in tune with the surrounding magnetic field. In mystic or spiritual language, we say that a man who has committed a sin comes and confesses in the house of the Lord and the Lord accepts his prayers and blesses him to the light.

He again starts living in a bountiful world. The two explanations are exactly the same. In this modern world, when there is a problem, people go to the psychiatrist who drinks coffee and has the patience to listen to them and to make them talk. Then, through his experience, he tells them that they have to work out the whole thing, cautiously. By charging a couple of thousand dollars, the psychiatrist makes the guy alert to the idea that he has to stop somewhere and solve his own problem. He has to put in an effort. This is what motivates him. It is not the psychiatrist; it is not the priest in the church. It is your acceptance of the environmental behaviors and the urge to look back to your basic origin and start understanding that you are the creative source and nucleus of the whole vibratory effect in which you live. The moment you understand this, you are alright, there's no problem. The moment you know you are you, the problem is solved. When you understand who and what you are, your radiance projects in the universal radiance and everything becomes creative around you. This confirmed relationship of responsiveness in consciousness between the finite self and the infinite self is the gift of kundalini.

What is the problem that arises between a father and son? Is there any father who wants to denounce his son? No. If he does denounce him, what forces him to? Some action of the son. If a father wants to accept his sort, what makes his son the most acceptable? Action. But action at what level? The action must be at the father's level of consciousness. If the father is a hunter and a fisherman, and the son goes and fishes and brings home a lot of fish, the father says, "Oh my, I'm impressed!" Suppose, instead, the son used to go for eight hours and get two fish. If he starts telling his father, "Fishing is no good. It is just killing the life in the ocean for no reason. Don't do it. You can't even create one fish but destroy as many as you can hook. How can you kill all those poor beautiful things in the ocean?" The father will get angry and say, "Okay. You get off my back and hit the road. Eat your own bread.

Get out of my house and keep going. I don't want to listen to you." He will react this way because he can't understand the son's point of view.

What is our understanding? It's our pattern of behavior. What is a pattern of behavior? It is the rate of frequency and the radiance of the psyche and the magnetic field in relationship to the universal psyche and magnetic force. If you can relate with that universal radiation so that the beam and frequency of projection is clear, then you have communicated with the universe and it will support you just as a happy father will support his son, his creation. This relationship of consciousness to the infinite consciousness is the one fundamental requirement of life and the aim of yoga.

There once was a businessman who wanted to find a man to manage his stores. He advertised. Everybody came with great experience and recommendations. The last interview was with a man who had no experience. The businessman said, "Why don't you have any recommendations?" He said, "Sir, if you want to recruit someone with a recommendation, you have already interviewed many. Just select one. But if you ever need a man, remember me and do call me. Thank you very much." He left smiling. The businessman started thinking. Is a manager a man, or is a man a manager? He sat on this problem for one week and finally came to a conclusion. A perfect manager may not be a man in the sense of activity. He discussed it with one of his friends. His friend said, "What are you talking about? That man just said I am a man, and you started believing him. What about his recommendations? These other people have already worked as managers of stores." The owner said, "They are managers of stores, but none of them could tell me that he is a man. I'd like to try this man." So he called him. He said, "Alright. You manage my store." The man said, "Sir, I have a problem. It is true I am a man. If you make a manager out of me then I'll manage the stores. My problem is that I am only a man, I am not yet a

manager." The businessman asked, "How can I train you in all those skills?" The man replied, "It is nothing. If you will just work for fifteen days as a manager, I will watch you and I will know." So the owner worked for fifteen days and this guy picked up everything. He was perfect. Sometime later they were sitting together and the owner asked, "I would like to understand something. How can you have all my confidence so that I trust you to do everything perfectly? You are not a very qualified man. Your only training was seeing me work for fifteen days." The new manager said, "Sir, one thing you must understand. I only know one thing: 'I am, I am.' My consciousness is very clear about the words 'I am, I am!' When anything bothers me, I tell myself one thing: 'I am, I am,' and I get to it. The moment you know you are you, there is no problem."

The basic unit of you is equal to your radiance plus your activity. That radiance is the mind and the activity is the gross. Let me express this in the mystic sense. When the soul opens up the heart, man becomes divine. You may say it any way you like. A man has to understand his existence in relationship to the universe. Whosoever understands this knows the truth. The whole world around you will be beautiful if you understand that you are you. In all walks of your life remember you are you. "I am, I am." That is the mantra. The kundalini and Kundalini Yoga are very natural elements that rapidly make you what you already are and bring you to the practical experience of Infinity.

Individual Harmony–Universal Harmony
by Yogi Bhajan, Ph.D.

These days there is a trend toward meditation in America, Western Europe and many other countries, but there is also much misunderstanding. I would like to go into depth on the subject. Our job is to teach it through the universities; to teach you what is what so that you can know the nature of what you are asking for. Then you can practice any way you like. Does anybody know what meditation is?

Audience: It would be like a silencing of the mind from everyday life and allowing the free flow of thought.

Audience: It is concentration.

Yogi Bhajan: That's part of it. Anybody else?

Audience: It is complete relaxation from regular hassles.

Yogi Bhajan: Come on, come on, everybody!

Audience: It's a new level of consciousness, a deeper level of consciousness. It's not exactly the same thing as our state of consciousness when we're doing something or when we have to relate to some function.

Audience: It is becoming receptive.

Yogi Bhajan: You all have one part or the other of meditation. Prayer is when the mind is one-pointed and man talks to Infinity. Meditation is when the mind becomes totally clean and receptive and Infinity talks to man. That is what meditation is. There are two levels of meditation. In one, this unit self talks to Infinity. In the other, Infinity talks to the unit. All the other

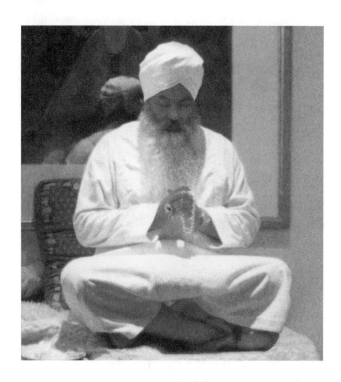

stages are preparations for meditation. You might have heard a lot these days about transcendental meditation and integral meditation and so many other meditations. If you want to sell mustard seed, you may call it yellow mustard, Sun Valley mustard seed, California mustard seed, Wisconsin mustard seed, or New York mustard seed; but the mustard seed is still a mustard seed. Meditation was labeled with many different names.

Similarly in yoga, the techniques to raise the kundalini were all different, so they were given different names; but they all have the same end. Hatha Yoga has the same end, which is to raise the kundalini in a person. Raja Yoga also has the same end. Bhakti, Shakti, Gyan, Karma Yoga—they all have the same end: They all want to raise the dormant power of infinity in man. That's all. There is a small difference. Suppose you want to go to San Francisco [from Los Angeles]. You can take Highway 1 or I-5, or an aircraft or a railway line, or go on a truck or hitchhike. The purpose is to reach San Francisco. By foot you can make it in two months or a month or twenty days; hitchhiking takes two days; a railway line takes 1 or 2 days; a car takes 8 to 10 hours; an aircraft will take you 45 minutes. Highway 1 will take you 10 hours; I-5 will take you 6½ hours. It is true that man has an infinite power which he can connect with through the techniques of yoga. There are different yogas around, different ways to go. Some take 30 years to practice while others take 30 days. The difference is only in time and technique.

The best way to meditate is in a creative meditation. The logic behind this is that the mind is mostly tuned to the intellect. The intellect starts giving thoughts and more thoughts, which relate to your emotion and temperament. They become desires, and desire then directs the body to create a creativity to earn the object or goal. This creativity is a practical experience in life.

Once I decided to rent a building. My staff said, "No, we want to have a permanent address. We don't want to rent. We will have to move, then later we will have to move again, etc." God sent us a person who found this property on Preuss Road, so I bought it. Once we bought it, everything went into it. We creatively thought about it and acted on it. Our one concern became, "What is the best atmosphere, what are the best circumstances, and in what way are they creative?" We put our whole energy into it in a very well-balanced manner. The result is this creative place and atmosphere we are teaching in tonight.

You can't live without meditation. Imagination and activity get blended to affect the focusing of the personality. That's what meditation is. You relate your unit activity toward your word of infinity. The question is: Are you creative or uncreative? That will decide the trend of your life. If you just sit for twenty minutes

and close yourself, that's not meditation. That is an effort, an attempt to prepare yourself for meditation. It is a preparation, not a complete result. Meditation is the creativity and activity which relates your existence to the existence of the cosmos. It is individual harmony in relationship to universal harmony.

When you come into contact with a living identity and remember infinity—that is God. When you meet a good man and you feel fulfilled—that is divine. Whenever you meet a living existence that enables you to expand to infinity in consciousness, you experience God. God is not a man. God is three letters, G–O–D: these represent the generating principle, the organizing principle, and the destroying principle. They took the first letter from each of these three words and made one word: GOD. The Hindus speak of Brahma, the god who gives birth; Vishnu, the god who sustains; and Shiva, the god who destroys. The Hindus worship them in idols; we have one word, GOD, which represents the same thing.

All churches and temples, synagogues and holy places are holy because the whole community can get together and relate together in unity unto infinity. That is why they are beautiful. Otherwise they have no purpose. They are places of creativity through divine meditation.

Audience: Well I get confused when you say . . .

Yogi Bhajan: First of all, remember that when you say, "I get confused," you are creating a vibration which confuses you. Don't use negative words. That is an uncreative meditation through a creative faculty. Three phrases you should never use: "I am confused," "I don't know," "I can't do it."

There are two parallel tendencies in a person: the urge to suicide and the urge to live. The higher mind runs on the living tendencies and does not go along with the suicidal tendencies. I feel it is my right to live because I have been created by the Infinity that is a Creator. Which tendency prevails depends on which you choose through your meditation and your words. Without creative meditation, a man will feel burdened. The law of detachment does not become functional for a man if he is not creative. Remember this law. It is the secret of spirituality which I'm explaining. Creative meditation is meditation in activity which links you with Infinity.

Detachment does not mean that you wear a loin cloth and carry a begging bowl and are detached from this world. Detachment comes from creative activity. If you only create a few things, you will feel attached to them. If you are constantly creating, you will feel free. You have been involved in many affairs and you have learned about failure and success. This has brought you to a state of attachment which will limit you. God has not made any person to limit himself. Man is not born to be limited. Death and life mean nothing to those who live moment–to–moment, in happiness, joy and creativity.

Audience: Can you be detached from your own emotions?

Why should you be detached from your emotions? You don't have to get rid of emotions and you don't have to have them either. You can just watch them. Let the emotion come. Let the emotion go. What comes should go. It is not emotions that prove you're alive. The way to find that out is to check your nose. If the breath goes in and out, then you are still alive.

You want to feel, I know. But has it ever occurred to you that you are so beautiful that the whole universe wants to tell you? Once you realize that you are invaluable, you don't have to make value judgments. Values come from attachment. We put a price on each

other because of our limited self; otherwise, each one is priceless. Where is the limit of a person? His limit is in his attachment. Man is basically unlimited because his soul is unlimited. Man is basically unlimited because his mind is unlimited. This structure is limited but it is priceless. Nobody can manufacture anything like this. Creative meditation uses this structure in relation to the cosmos.

Do you know how things go on around this Earth? Science may find within a thousand years that the life–sound comes from the sun. That sound is the existence of the atom. Then they will find that we have within us a little sun. Therefore our existence is also the existence of the atom, and we make an impact on the universe just as it makes an impact on us. Every person thinks he knows everything without knowing what he knows. That is the mystery of life. We all know how successful we can be without knowing what success is. Does anybody know what success is?

Audience: The opposite of failure.

Yogi Bhajan: That is the right answer. You think that riches make you successful? I can give you telephone numbers of rich people who have got plenty of money and comfort. All they want is to be able to sleep. If you think power is success, I can also give you the numbers of powerful people. They think they are God if they can get time to eat or relax. It is a strange, strange world. I have everything which a normal American can think of, but I am still free.

We get so attached to things! If it is the rainy season, we get upset, as if we were paper and were going to melt. If it is summer, we get upset. If there were no summer, what would happen? Somebody was saying to me, "Oh, spring is coming. There will be hay fever." The moment spring comes people start thinking of hay fever. Nobody thinks of the beauty of spring when everything blooms.

19

When your mind is totally creative, nothing will come to you without a purpose. Nothing will happen to you without a purpose. Nothing will bind you with attachment to the cycle of worry and pain. Success will be a subconscious habit. Creative meditation is when the creative mind accepts itself as part of the universe. The whole universe then becomes part of you. A creative mind knows that wherever he is, he can be creative. When you become a part of the universe, the universe becomes part of you. That is creative meditation: minute–to–minute, time–to–time, being–to–being, place–to–place, and breath–to–breath. Each breath which goes in you goes in under the divine will and it comes out under divine will. So what are you worried about?

Who among you has the power to breathe? What is breath to you? It means life. It is life. What is life? Life is a bindu, a point. It has been vitalized and energized to go in the longitude and latitude, on the orbit of time, to a specific length. Its glow depends on its own vibration. If your vibration is universal, you've become a universal man. If it's national, you've become a national man. If you have a city vibration, you are a city man. If you are little, you are a little man. You can decide. That much is your choice. As you expand your mind, you expand. As you limit your mind, you are limited.

Life is not under your control and the mind is not obedient, but there is something the mind does obey. That is the rate of the breath. The mind knows if its body is not going to have breath, the mind will have nothing to do with the body. When the breath is long and deep and slow, the mind is constant and one-pointed. When the breath is heavy, quick, and shallow, the mind is scattered. You normally breathe 15 breaths a minute. If you can train yourself to breathe 8 breaths per minute, you can have your temper and your projection under control. It is the most creative meditation you can do. Expand the mind and become part of the whole cosmic process. Become creative, unattached, and carefree—but not careless. Take meditation to heart, as a golden path to Infinity, which must be experienced in practical activity each day.

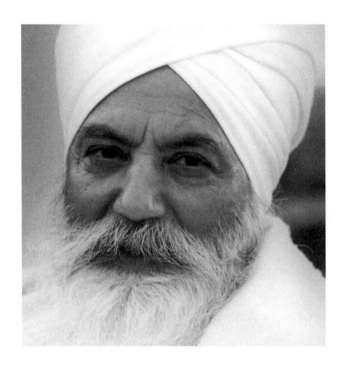

Take meditation to heart,
as a golden path to Infinity,
which must be experienced
in practical activity each day.

–Yogi Bhahan

*Looking Forward and Looking Back
by Gurucharan Singh Khalsa, Ph.D.*

The world is crossing a threshold. Our civilization is changing its form as radically as ice changes to water and water changes to vapor. We are the same, but our consciousness, our energy patterns, our capacity to perceive, our social relationships, our technological sophistication and spiritual reality are all shifting. Yogi Bhajan foreshadowed this fundamental change in our global civilization and in our concept of ourselves as human beings in 1969 when he began to teach Kundalini Yoga—The Yoga of Awareness—to Western audiences and to the world. At that time he called the impending change "the dawning of the Aquarian Age." He described its characteristics as well as the capacities and caliber we would each need to excel in this new environment. He guided us through the nature of the ego, the structure of the mind, the hidden energies within the body and the testable reality of our experience as a conscious soul. He gave us the tools we would need to awaken our awareness, cultivate our compassion, elevate our consciousness and prosper on this path he declared to be our birthright—the healthy, happy, and holy way of life (3HO).

The foundation for human excellence—to live a meaningful and effective life in this new Age—is the practice of sadhana. What is sadhana? A personal self-discipline to experience and realize your Self, master the mind, and soften the ego's dominance over our habits, emotions and thoughts. Develop a regular sadhana and you take control of your life. Develop a deep sadhana and you open the doors of experience. Commit to meet your higher Self each morning and your decisions and your life become original; your life will bear the signature of your soul; your radiance will

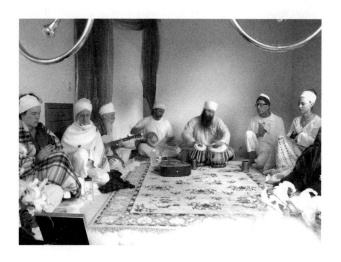

express the meaningful intimacy of the Infinite in each moment. Immerse yourself in the joy of victory that comes from starting each day with a powerful sadhana and every challenge becomes an opportunity.

In this essay, I will endeavor to distill the essence of a good sadhana. What is it? What are its goals? How does it work? What are its effects? What are the obstacles to a personal practice? What are the first steps? And what are the stages we go through as we practice? What are examples of great sadhanas you can practice and master?

What is Sadhana?

Sadhana is a self-discipline by which we energize and balance the body and clear the mind and subconscious. Sadhana is also a spiritual practice in which we confront the tendencies of our mind and ego and out of love invite in the dimensions of our soul, spirit and intuition. Sadhana, in its essence, is a process of refinement, development and mastery. In this sense, there are unlimited forms and techniques used to create the experiences that we call sadhana. Each tradition of mastery in yoga, martial arts or any performing art has explored and refined techniques that create the most progress for an individual in the least time toward the goals of that tradition. In Kundalini Yoga as taught by Yogi Bhajan®, the goal is awareness, caliber, character, consciousness and the ability to live as a fulfilled and unique human being. How can we manifest our human excellence? How can we live to be healthy, happy and holy? Sadhana.

The mother, and queen, of all sadhanas is morning sadhana. Morning sadhana is done in the 2½ hours before the rise of the sun. Wisdom traditions of all types have discovered the special qualities of this early time of the morning, these ambrosial hours, in which we can determine our reality and separate ourselves from fantasies, illusions, and even delusions, the denizens of our subconscious. A sadhana can also be a special period of time where we focus on the practice of one technique—a kriya, meditation, or mantra— for 40, 90, 120, or 1000 days, or a lifetime. It might last 11 minutes, 31 minutes, 2½ hours, or more. The time commitment will depend on the purpose and the technique used.

A sadhana can also help make unconscious habits conscious. It might entail a conscious fast in which we confront our choices around food and the way in which we nurture and accept the gift of our body. Some sadhanas take advantage of the day's rhythms. A meditation may occur as the sun sets, or at a full moon, or during a special time of year in which we want to take advantage of special cyclical qualities in the seasons. In addition to the long commitments, a sadhana can also be intensive, focused on for only a few days.

Think of the morning sadhana as the foundation for all sadhanas. With the morning sadhana well-established in your mind and heart and habits, you may cultivate a variety of sadhanas yourself, or under the guidance of a qualified teacher, in order to enhance your practice, balance a particular aspect of your mind, or adjust the qualities in yourself that you are working on. The goals and the primary nature of sadhana as well as its many facets and effects were described eloquently by Yogi Bhajan.

Sadhana is self-enrichment. It is not something which is done to please somebody or to gain something. Sadhana is a personal process in which you bring out your personal best.   —Yogi Bhajan, July 16, 1982

Your real sadhana, a spiritually powerful sadhana, arises from the inside. It wells up from the heart with the motivation of love and flowers naturally into discipline. A sadhana may involve many efforts depending on the technique that you use. You may sit in stillness for many hours; you may exercise with vigor and rhythm; or you may go beyond the constraints of your mind and its thoughts as you merge into the repeated sounds of a mantra or prayer. But all these efforts are truly effortless efforts. The goal of the sadhana is the awakening of the Self that is the soul. It is the experience of your consciousness and your purpose in this moment. It is not done to control the world, win the lottery, perfect your personality or attain any recognition. It is for self-enrichment. And that Self that you open to in sadhana has no bounds; it is a gift of the Creator that is beyond form and time; it is infinite. Sadhana brings this infinite dimension of ourselves and our existence into our daily experience.

Sadhana is practical. It brings us into an intimate alignment with the reality of who we are: as a creature of the Creator and as a human being. Each of us must deal daily with our fluctuating levels of energy. If we know how to tap into the source of energy within ourselves and our stillness, we can act consciously in every moment and not just react to the shifting tides that beset us from within and without. Knowing how to shift gears and adjust our level of energy helps us to act in a way that represents who we truly are.

Why do we get up in the morning? Because we have to face the whole day and we cannot face the day without a constant level of energy.

People love you for three things: wisdom, commitment and consistency. If you think anybody loves you without these qualities you are the biggest idiot ever born in a human body.

Wisdom is the intuitiveness that allows you to give the right answer by listening within the question that is asked. For every question there is an answer in it. It comes to you already complete, as a Cycle of Verbalization.

Commitment is the ability for your whole self to sustain its status in the projected reality of your actions. Then people can trust you. Otherwise it is like building a cozy bungalow on the top of a volcano. If you act like an earthquake or volcano, who will build upon you?

Consistency is steadiness through time. If you say as a question "I want to know that I know," this is the question that comes from the desire for consistency. The answer within the question is "And what I know is known."

Sadhana gives us sensitivity to know, to feel and to touch. It gives us intuition to touch reality. The methods are three fold: japa, tapa and sanjam. Japa is repetition. Tapa is the heat of central impulsation. Sanjam is merger through simran—meditation on a very slow, conscious breath. Women in Training XII, *1987, p. 41*

What is sin? Sin is a fluctuation in the flow of spirit like the high and low tide. When a person is in very low spirits, he cannot represent the flow of his spirit. The tide is out and nobody can come into dock. This is the biggest sin of all. When the tide is in, you are bright, beautiful,

and wonderful. You have the spirit to match up to everything.

How can you keep the tide in? How can you maintain your depth? I can tell you the answer in one word: sadhana. I can lecture without end. But I have already told you the truth. There is no other truth. All situations can totally be taken care of if a person decides to do sadhana every morning. Women in Training V, *1980, p. 119*

The experience we cultivate in a regular sadhana builds our capacity to be flexible, conscious and consistent. Yogi Bhajan would call that capacity our caliber, character and grit. No intellectual knowledge can give that to us. No committed belief or earnest enthusiasm can build the foundation of self-trust and character necessary. We must have experience. The pathway to character and spiritual abundance—the way to give ourselves that experience—is sadhana.

Sadhana is a test of self-grit. If your sadhana is more important than your neurosis, you are fine. If your neurosis is more important than your sadhana you are not. Doesn't matter how saintly you are, nobody wants to get up in the ambrosial hours. Why you still do it is a mystery. At that time, between 3 and 6 o'clock, the rays of the sun pass at 60 degrees to the earth and you want to feel relaxed. You take a cold shower, wake-up and meditate. Why do you repeat the mantra hundreds of times? To create a stamina, an absolute mental stamina—without which there is no chance for life to be smooth. If somebody refuses to exercise, nobody can force him. But at that one moment in life when that person needs physical stamina, it won't be there. Sadhana is what your mental stamina requires. Love is what your spiritual stamina requires. —Yogi Bhajan, January 22, 1991

Sadhana is a process to refine the human awareness, to burn off the old patterns and to clean out the subconscious. Women in Training XII, *1987, p. 134*

Sadhana brings us to reality. Is there any unreality in us? No. We are as real as God is.

—Yogi Bhajan, March 22, 1983

As we gain stamina through sadhana, we are infused with a quality of stillness, a presence and neutrality that is known as nonattachment. Instead of chasing our thoughts or reacting to our emotions, we become present. From this profound stillness that we call *shuniya*, we can recognize ourselves, love ourselves, and accept and love the entire creation. From this place of stillness, we can release our inner tension and expand our sensitivity and perception so that everything comes through clearly. Our intuition begins to serve the purpose of our soul. This beautiful and empowered state is not automatic. It requires work—the hard work of sadhana. It requires commitment. Yet, it is not something that we can force. Much like preparing one's house for a special guest, we cannot force the guest into our home; but we can make the house so attractive, so cozy and so full of love that the guest cannot help but come for a visit.

We have to clean out the patterns and reactions of our subconscious. As we do, the reality of who we are and the reality of the infinite spirit that already exists within us, and everywhere, becomes clear. Being awakened is simple, practical and quintessentially human.

We do sadhana selfishly. We don't do sadhana to please God. Take it out of your mind. I have never done sadhana with an absolute feeling that I'll please God, or I'll have good luck or my tomorrow will be fine. I have absolutely no such understanding—zero percent. I do sadhana so that when I'm put on the frying pan, I'll cry just a little less than anybody else. That's all. I'll have maybe 10% more chance of self-control than another person. Sadhana has nothing to do with God, the Almighty or anything else. Sadhana is "I take a bath, because I don't want to stink. I do sadhana, because I don't

want to go out of control." At that time I have to change my—what you call it?—Gears! If I have done sadhana, I can change them through the whole day.

—Yogi Bhajan, February 22, 1990

Sadhana gives you grace. Sadhana gives you fearlessness. Sadhana gives you self. Sadhana gives you denomination, domination, projection, polarity combination, equilibrium, respectability, totality, internal and external self-knowledge. Sadhana gives you purity; and it gives you divinity, dignity, and grace. It gives you radiance, it gives you pranic Shakti, and it gives you auric Shakti.

It makes you like a special metal that is always shining, yet unseen. You become a metallically living grace. In Punjabi language we say, "loh" which means iron. But loh also means that which can absorb the entire heat. When you go to the house of Guru Ram Das they put a big sheet of iron on which they cook chapattis; that is called loh. The quality you gain is called "sarb loh." Sarb loh does not mean a person who wears all iron (in malas, weapons and jewelry) about himself. That is a misappropriation of the reality of what is meant. Sarb loh means that loh which takes the entire coolness and heat of all the universe, and still remains neutral. A metallic grace.

That is what sadhana gives you. When you want to be bountiful, do sadhana. It makes you very attractive and shining. It is one thing you will find my dear, whether you belong to dharma or you don't belong to dharma. If you belong to a dharma, then fine. If you don't belong to a dharma, then you belong to karma. But somewhere the karma has to stop, dharma has to start, who will decide that?

Who will decide who you are? Who will decide? Because every time in your life one chance must come—one chance, just one chance—where you can be you for that one second, for that one moment. And that will only come to you through sadhana. Sadhana is nothing but the death of karma, all wrong things, all misfortunes, all bad things, all bad lucks, all sins are evaporated during the period of sadhana.

Sadhana eliminates and neutralizes misfortune, tragedies, bad luck, non-reality, and all sickness. The direction of your life is not your reactions to life. The direction of life is in the resurrection of life. . . .
        —Yogi Bhajan, July 30, 1980

The 3HO way of life—as a Kundalini Yogi and an awakened human—revolves around sadhana. It is the hub of our lives; the fulcrum which elevates us; and the axis on which we spin. Sadhana is a challenge, to our habits and to our mind, through which we can experience victory and the full flowering of our Self and our Soul, initiating every action from the full faith and reality of our heart. We can then embrace the reality of each moment and the vastness that accompanies us seamlessly through our life. When we live that, we realize our uniqueness even as we merge with the One in all.

Yogi Bhajan was very clear about this experience, within his own life and in the traditions of Kundalini Yoga. He shared the techniques of how to have an extraordinary sadhana and he gave us the challenge through which we can invite in and receive that special guest—our spirit.

I am not the way you want to look at me; I am the way I am. I just do because I have to do. Because what I have learned in my life is that duty is beauty—there is nothing to match it. Victory is victory—there's nothing to substitute it. Character is divine—there is nothing equal to it. Equilibrium is an experience which you cannot do any other way but through sadhana; there is no other way to it.

Life has a category and in this category there's a 'fantasticness.' Life is a fantastic thing! Our commitment is a most fantastic thing. Then our living to that commitment is the ultimate fantastic thing. That is the 3HO way of life: healthy, happy, holy. First commit, then live to the commitment and then experience the commitment. There's no other way to be happy.
        —Yogi Bhajan, September 9, 1980

The Spiritual Dimension of Sadhana

What about the spiritual dimension of sadhana, how should we think about that? Yogi Bhajan was fond of saying that we are spiritual beings having a human experience. So our job as human beings is not to search out the spirit and try to find God. Nor is it to cultivate extraordinary experiences, miracles, or special powers *(siddhis)* because the universe itself is the most extraordinary miracle that is or can be. Rather, our task is to recognize God, recognize our self as a human being, and recognize the opportunity in each moment to serve, to be compassionate and to be kind.

What blocks our capacity to recognize God and the Infinite within our self? The noise and habits of the mind, our ego and its attachments and fears, and our assumption that God is something outside of ourselves, something separate, distant or accessible to only a few. In this Aquarian Age, we must find the experience of the divine within us, connect to our own higher Self and deliver that reality in the actions and attitudes of our life.

The purpose of sadhana is to arrive at the moment when we go beyond our ego and its limitations. Morning sadhana—in the *amrit vela*—is a special time, a time when we can receive the blessings and the grace of teachers from every Age, beyond the limits of the here and now. It is a time when we can sit before the altar of our own consciousness and have the opportunity to clean up our inner world before we engage in the outer world—our jobs, our families, our responsibilities. We become still. We surrender our ego, our emotions and our reactions to the clarity, compassion and commitment that resides in our heart. That is our higher Self. As we attain this clarity and stillness, automatically, without effort, the perception of God in All comes to us. We experience this insight uniquely, according to our *tattvas*, qualities and karma, but the unity of the consciousness is available to each of us.

Sadhana, in itself, is a universal process. When we drop our constraints, fears, and attachments to the mind's concepts of that which is actually beyond the mind, we find the unlimited presence of God within us and all around us. We realize our natural connection to things—beyond our conditioning and beliefs about ourselves. This is the purpose of all religions and wisdom paths—the singular experience of oneness with all, to know that we're not alone. Sadhana simply opens the window. Sadhana gives us the clarity to see and enjoy our human experience and our connection to everything in creation—through spirit—no matter what path we have been placed on by the hands of grace.

This concept of sadhana—as a universal process—is why yoga is not a religion. Yogi Bhajan called himself a spiritual scientist. He shared the techniques and traditions that give us the ability to optimize ourselves as human beings.

The first act of surrendering to God is to live as He has made you. The second act of surrendering to God is to maintain what hair God has given you on the crown of your head. The third act of sacrifice is to meditate on the five primal sounds (Sa-Ta-Na-Ma) in the morning and praise the Lord before the sun rises. Teachings of Yogi Bhajan, p. 179

Sadhana is the foundation on which the House of Consciousness is built. Its value is universal and its practice is timeless. In this cusp period, the transition to the Aquarian Age from the Piscean Age, sadhana takes on special import. This changing of the Age means the end of adolescence for humankind. Every adolescent experiences growing pains and periods of struggle to realize and manifest their adult potentials. The same is true in the history of our evolving consciousness. Conditions are changing both within us and around us. We are globalizing. We are connected to everyone, everywhere. Everything is known, or will be known. We must have the grace and consciousness to encounter and uplift people from all faiths, all religions—even those who believe in nothing.

It is now easy to interconnect electronically or by travel to any place and with any person on the globe. For thousands of years people traveled around the globe, but it was infrequent and done only by a privileged few. We lived village-by-village. Our scope and need for tolerance and understanding had a radius of 15 to 50 miles. Explorers and mystics expanded our awareness of the 'other,' of faraway places and ideas. Now, all ideas, people and beliefs come to us no matter where we are. How should we adapt and thrive in this time of intense and creative interconnection? We must become conscious of our self within our self so that we can see and feel each other clearly. We must act with both grace and effectiveness; we must strive to understand each other and use harmonious, conscious communication to bridge our differences.

The change within each of us, individually, is equally profound. Our sense of who we are, our responsibilities and our potential are shifting radically. Instead of viewing ourselves as a small piece of dust, glorified with grand delusions, we shall see ourselves as an intricate, but finite, physical vessel linked to an infinite source of universal consciousness and energy. The tide of our inner evolution will wash away the old concepts of individuality and awaken our intuition and our trust. The meaning and stability of life will emerge from the harmony between the individual psyche and the universal psyche. We will not rely on institutions in the same way. We will strive to create lifestyles which unleash our highest potential as we thrive in our individual, global and cosmic consciousness.

The traditional astrological symbol for the Age of Aquarius is the bearer of truth. Its motto is "I know, therefore I believe." The old way of knowing was "I believe, therefore I know." Now and in the future, people will increasingly demand a practical, personal experience to verify the ancient spiritual truths. Nothing will be accepted without being tested and beliefs without experience will carry no weight. The test of that experience will not be in our membership or creeds but in how well we can deliver consciousness and caliber through our actions. To build an authentic experience within yourself, be it from grace or grit, requires constant practice and a commitment to your higher consciousness—sadhana. Such a profound transformation of consciousness may bring periods of turmoil and creative chaos, especially in the ways we interact with one another, our lifestyles, our choices, and our allegiances. Those locked into the old consciousness may put up a great fight to retain the old ways, even as they slip away like sand in the surf, churned into the depths by relentless waves of change, driven by forces unseen.

The foundation of these new lifestyles will be sadhana: a disciplined practice to integrate body, mind, and spirit. The techniques taught by Yogi Bhajan and the lifestyle and discipline of Kundalini Yoga offer each of us an effective and efficient way to realize the potential of each person. The first teaching of this lifestyle is to rise before dawn every day and do a sadhana. It cannot be overemphasized. It should not be overlooked.

The following discussion offers guidelines for a powerful personal practice and an effective group sadhana. It will help you not to just do sadhana but to be sadhana with each breath.

Process and Progress in Sadhana
Sadhana. Aradhana and Prabhupati

Sadhana

The practice of sadhana is a continuous refinement of the self and it has a natural progression through stages. The three classical stages that one goes through are *sadhana, aradhana,* and *prabhupati.* Roughly translated, these mean discipline, attitude, and aptitude or mastery. Note that the word "sadhana" is used in two ways: Sadhana is the overall practice, with all its stages; *and* it is one of the three stages that we pass through as we master ourselves and our Sadhana. "Sadhana" and "sadhana." The three steps are inseparable, each supporting and developing the others.

Sadhana refines the quality and develops the characteristics of our consciousness as human beings: The stages reflect steps on the way toward the mastery of our habits; the techniques used in sadhana lessen the sway of our ego; the process of refinement reflects the crystallization of our awareness and caliber. Sadhana is a process to refine human awareness, burn off the old patterns and clean out the subconscious. Yogi Bhajan called this refinement, self-crystallization. The ideal is to make your mind a diamond–mind, with a flawless gem quality worthy of the greatest museums. He describes this self-crystallization process:

You cannot achieve in life, you cannot crystallize your self in your life without discipline. There are scientific terms we are all familiar with: distillation, sublimation and crystallization. Distillation is to purify. That is the everyday sadhana that we do. It is a distillation to remove impurities like a filter. Sublimation is next. It is more subtle and complete. It is the transformation of something to a higher state of energy. Sublimation leaves all deeply imbedded impurity behind. It is just like taking a block of sulfur and heating it up so all the sulfur becomes a vapor and the impurities remain below. That is what kirtan is—sublimation through word. Last is crystallization. When purification is advanced, you collect the substance around a single pure crystal. Even that process of refinement has steps and stages. The seed must be perfect. The temperature and environments must be constant. If all things are held steady in perfection then you get a perfect gem. Usually the resulting crystallization has four levels of quality. The most familiar is "opaque" or raw rock form. It is the right substance, but it may be covered on the surface and have many flaws in its structure so it does not have its full strength or transparency. The next quality is "semi-precious gem." It is clearer, without a surface cover and a few flaws. The third quality is the "gem state." That is beautiful. It has few to no flaws and can carry clear light. The fourth quality is very rare indeed. It is flawless, with perfect structure and strength. That gem has a perfect cut in its facets and can reflect everything perfectly, with no distortion.

Women in Training XII, *1987, p. 134*

Crystallization is complete when what began as a goal-oriented effort becomes a spontaneous expression of joy, gratitude and love in a living discipline that arises from within our consciousness, seamlessly imbued in each moment, action by action. These stages are similar to the four stages referred to in Vedanta as waking, dreaming, deep sleep, and awakened sleep—*turiya*. The first is opaque and narrow, attached and self-concerned. The second is imaginative, elaborative and creative. The third is filled with stillness and the ability to know many things intuitively; one can leave the ego and perceive or heal without the limits of distance or time. The last state knows the Infinite in the finite form. It is dwelling in God, flowing with dharma, acting in synchrony and harmony with the flow of the greater Being and one's destiny. It is neutral and reflects all things accurately. It is intuition—immanent and embodied—in constant spontaneous creativity. This is only achieved by going through the three stages of practice: *sadhana, aradhana,* and finally, *prabhupati.*

The first step is daily sadhana, which we've defined in broader terms but here, we explore sadhana as expressed in personal practice. *Sadhana* means any practice of self-correction that provides the mind and body with a disciplined procedure to express the Infinite within one's self. It is a practice that aligns your cycles, patterns, and mental and emotional reactions so that they support your purpose, your values and your goals. It is a time each day to notice all the negative habits that lead you away from higher consciousness and to eliminate the desires underlying those habits one-by-one—step-by-step.

This is a conscious activity. It is not automatic. You consciously choose to wake up in the early hours of the morning instead of sleeping. You consciously exercise the body and exalt the Infinite in your heart with your voice and projected attitude. Each day is different. Each day—you are different. Every 72 hours most of the cells of your body change. Sickness comes and goes. Motivation waxes and wanes. But through all the flux of life, through all the fickle reactions of our emotions, through all the palpitations of our unsure heart, and through the maelstrom of our thoughts and ideas, we consciously choose to maintain a constant and regular practice. By this commitment we establish a priority in life above all the changes: We choose to exalt the Infinite Universal Self and to develop our human, finite self as a channel to express our subtle and unlimited nature.

The yogic scriptures require at least 2½ hours of sadhana before the rising of the sun. In this way, you dedicate at least one-tenth of each day to refining your consciousness, maintaining your vitality and connecting to the sacred dimension of yourself and God. In these early ambrosial hours, the *prana*, the basic life force of consciousness, concentrates and physical cleansing is more easily accomplished than in the later hours of the day. It is a tranquil time when few people are awake and busy, so the clutter and bustle of daily activities will not distract or interfere with your practice and clarity.

Though many things may challenge the constancy or depth of your early morning sadhana, as you conquer each one, you will build your will power, your confidence, and the ability to creatively and consciously beam your mind. This constant practice of stillness, awareness and readiness infuses your life with sensitivity to the natural rhythms of your body and to the fertile dance of each moment. This is no small accomplishment. If at the same time each day, you attune all your mental and physical rhythms to each other, then no part of yourself will be out of step with any other part of yourself. The entire day flows better. Doing a sadhana at the same time each day helps you master it quickly because your body and mind use that regularity to anchor your consciousness. Regular practice is part of the art of learning the enterprise of self-mastery. Learning theory has shown that if you practice a particular task at the same time each day, you will learn it more efficiently. Therefore, if you practice meditation at the same time every day, it becomes easier and easier.

In meditation, you clean the subconscious mind of its fears and anxieties and in turn release reservoirs of consciousness and energy—you renew yourself. You cultivate new habits: allowing your awareness to guide you; no longer chasing the thoughts and reactions of your mind; practicing neutrality and flexibility. As each fear comes up, look at it with neutrality and your instinctual and learned fears will release their power over you. You become flexible; you break the rigid automatic behaviors induced by anxiety, fear and depression. Most of our fears were learned at a particular time of day and anchored to specific circumstances or thoughts. These fears tend to occur most intensely when triggered by similar circumstances, time periods or thought patterns that initiated them in the first place. By meditating during early morning sadhana, we slowly process these anxieties consciously, while under our control rather than becoming subject to their reactions as they arise on their own in our daily life.

Normally you react to anxieties on their time and on their conditions. Your subconscious reactions and emotions crowd out your awareness and the reality of the moment. In meditation, these old fears come to you on your time and under your conditions. Because your practice is at the same time each day, it becomes increasingly easier to process and redirect the fears as you establish and dwell in the clarity of your own consciousness. Eventually the mind is cleared—the clouds of fear, anger, depression and fantasy part and the light and power of creative consciousness begins to reveal itself.

Aradhana

Gradually your sadhana practice develops into an attitude of life and a consistent habit—*aradhana*, the second stage of discipline. After practicing a regular sadhana for some time, the teachings and the consciousness they instill begin to seep into the deeper recesses of the mind. It takes time for a conscious action or habit to permeate the subconscious and finally command the unconscious. To master a new habit traditionally takes 40 days of consistent action. You begin to sense the results of your actions and benefit from new perceptions, energy and behaviors. To stabilize it across all conditions may take 90 days. To make it flow spontaneously as you focus on other things may take 120 days. To penetrate past old blocks, fears and other habits could take a much more sustained effort—often years. It depends on the individual, the intensity and consistency of effort, and the starting conditions.

Once you've reached this stage, the efforts which you consciously planted have grown roots, and the offshoots are able to stand on their own. The subconscious mind finally gets the message. It understands that you are sincere; that meditation is a priority; that every day, at this time, you wake up automatically, ready for sadhana. It realizes that it is as necessary as breathing; you do it no matter what else is happening in your life. The subconscious begins to support you and sadhana begins to feel effortless. The subconscious, which directs about 85% of our activities and responses, has now acquired a habit—a habit to support your growth in consciousness and awareness through the practice of sadhana.

In the beginning, the willful, conscious effort to do sadhana may seem like a negative activity. It imposes a discipline at the cost of some other activities—like sleep! It confronts you with every possible impediment in your attempts to be regular. But as sadhana grows into *aradhana*, victory, confidence and gratitude come from the struggle. You have established a procedure that awakens the desire of your higher mind to connect with the universal self. During *aradhana*, the mind becomes more active and sadhana more profound in its subconscious clearing. If you find resistance or challenge in this stage, its source shifts. It is no longer from the flux of the mind or external impediments. Instead you now confront a basic question: Are you willing to act and think in your highest consciousness, or do you want to hang on to your old identity even longer? Do you continue to take your cue from the feelings and familiar emotions of your ego or do you begin to act from the sensitivity of your consciousness? Do you identify with your ego? Do you follow your personality? Or, do you identify with your heart and soul and use your personality and your ego to serve your destiny? If you choose the higher self, then sadhana becomes a joy and you leap up each morning to meet it. If you put off the decision, you vacillate: first motivated, then unmotivated. You exaggerate: feel more tired or sick than you may be in order to avoid getting up. You sleep: whenever you start to meditate, you may doze off in an attempt to avoid the profound transformation that comes with this commitment to your self. These are common pitfalls at this stage of development.

However, the more serious pitfall at this stage is the feeling that you have "made it." Since the physical habit became firmly established, perhaps you have become lax in the mental discipline of beaming the mind to the Infinite. It is just like climbing a mountain: When you reach a high plateau, your impulse is to camp and look at the valley below, dine on succulent berries and rest from the strenuous climb. But waiting too long makes the muscles slack and soon you may even forget why you wanted to climb to the top in the first place when you are so comfortable here. You know the rest of the climb is harder, narrower, and colder than what you have already experienced. So you resist the last step.

So it is in our climb toward self-realization and personal excellence. When we have practiced enough to confirm an attitude, we relax. We make it to sadhana, but fall asleep. We will chant the *Nam*—the sacred sounds and names of God—but sometimes feel the words are just mechanical sounds without meaning because we have lost touch with our initial motivation and intention. This is normal. It is part of the subconscious reorganization that affects motivation and intention. At some point in this, you may feel absolutely no motivation to continue. It is at such moments that the regular habit and the commitment to doing sadhana support you; in fact, it is essential. Your dutiful commitment and your love of the *Nam* may become your only reasons for continuing. If you are constant through this dark time, you can tap new sources of energy and strength within yourself. As your feelings clarify and begin to support you, you will build reliance directly on the Infinite and never need to rely on a finite motivation or structure for your sense of self, or your purpose, or your power to act creatively.

Prabhupati

The final stage, *prabhupati*, represents opening and attunement to the super-consciousness. Once *aradhana* has thoroughly cleaned the subconscious and set your motivation to know, merge, and use the Infinite as your base, you enter into *prabhupati*, or Mastery of God. This is the state of neutrality. Your motivation dwells in the neutral mind. It is neither for nor against anything. It expresses only what is. It experiences neither attachment nor aversion, only being. No finite thing motivates you: money, fame, sex, or personal advancement do not determine your actions. You cease to be manipulated by things. Most of us are so attached to our possessions, and our hopes, and even our fears, that we cannot, with each breath, act creatively and freely in the highest consciousness. Instead, we compromise our potential, our future, to possess our past. But in this neutral state, you can sense the Infinite in all things and nothing motivates you beyond this experience of the Infinite itself. You become free of causation and your motivation comes only from the center of your being—from within.

In this stage, the conscious mind has merged beyond the subconscious mind into the super-conscious mind, and there is no conflict with your personality. You are not divided by the conflicts that every personality has due to its dynamic structure. Everything is experienced as harmony. Even if the gross outward circumstance seems challenging or disastrous, you sense more. You accept more. You can feel more of the pain, and more of the joy, of every person across the entire globe, but still you rest in the neutral mind— sublime, pragmatic and subtle. Intention and action merge seamlessly into spontaneous readiness to accept what is and to do what is original and organic to your awareness and values. This is Mastery of God— *prabhupati*. In this concept there is not a God external or separate from you. The Infinite is intimate; you dwell in God and God in you. Your sacred higher Self manifests in every thought, feeling and cell of your body. You embody godliness through your kindness, compassion and caliber. *Prabhupati* means that you have cultivated faith in your own mind; you trust that every action is from your being, beyond mind. The unseen flows comfortably with the seen.

Soul and mind reconcile into dharma. You drop the attachment to a single thought or belief as you invoke your consciousness, which exists beyond thoughts. This is the full awakening and integration of compassion into the personality. Compassion gives us the capacity to forgive the unforgivable. Normally, we do not see God in All; we see God in a few—people or actions we deem "good"—if at all. We love those we like instead of loving everyone—especially our enemies. To have true compassion, we must perceive and experience the subtle within us that is beyond mind, beyond form, that which gives rise to all forms and existence. To be compassionate we must learn to become zero; we must practice non-existence. We must dwell only in the sacred being of God and our own Infinity. Without that habit of stillness within our mind and ego, we get caught defending or prosecuting what we feel is good or bad, holy or unholy, and we lose the capacity for authentic love and compassion. We risk being religious without being spiritual; or its reverse. We need both—the free flow of the spirit manifest in disciplined, compassionate action.

The Law of Polarity

The Law of Polarity rules action and reaction throughout the cosmos. Everything must come to balance. What you give, you get. If you steal, the law of balance requires someone or something to steal from you. This provides an order to the world that we call karma—actions have an effect and a balance in the totality of life. Because these laws govern the flow of events in a normal life, the circumstances we live in function to teach us, to reflect our actions and the actions of others. By accepting and embracing each moment, we can begin to recognize our patterns as opportunities to change—to begin moving toward our destiny and not our fate. We can act from consciousness instead of reacting and, in so doing, align to the flow of "God's Will" or dharmic action that is free from the narrow constraints of ego or fear. This is the state of *prabhupati*. Those who act beyond the laws of time and polarity; those who act from intuition with authentic compassion; they are the exception. They are exceptional—beyond the law of karma.

Such an accomplished person, a *sadhu*, who has mastered *prabhupati* can forgive the thief, welcome the lost, and inspire the hopeless. This great one can plant in that dark heart the spark of inspiration that brings out the hidden potential of their infinite self and destiny.

The Story of Valmiki

Yogi Bhajan often recounted a story, told in many ways, that shows the power of this potential in each of us. This is the story of Valmiki who was to write the famous *Ramayana* (the story of Lord Rama) from the Hindu tradition:

Valmiki was separated from his parents when he was very young and was raised by a hunter and woodsman. He became skilled in hunting, killing and survival. Once he married and had many children, he could not support them well, so he took up highway robbery as his means. He was by profession a *dacoit*—a thief and a head-cutter—with an excellent reputation for efficiency and success. No one ever passed Valmiki's hiding spot without getting his head parted from his body and his coin placed in the head-cutter's pocket. For generations his whole family had been taught this skill. With diligent study, he became the best of all. People who knew of his reputation stayed away. Even the king's men did not challenge him.

On this particular day a traveling holy man, an un-

named *sadhu* (though some say it was Narada), who had not heard the stories walked by the robber's lair. Valmiki jumped him with raised sword and began to take everything from him, even his clothes. To his surprise, the saint kneeled with bowed head and thanked the thief slyly, "You are most generous to give me my day of liberation, kind thief. I have waited long to leave this physical body. Please hurry so I may join the Creator!" The thief never had a client who uttered such a strange plea. The *sadhu* did not have much money. He said to Valmiki, "there is not much, why take it?" He replied, "A little here and a little there adds up to a lot." The saint replied, "It is the same with karma and ill-action, a little here and a little there adds up to a lot and it ruins your life—its sinks your boat!"

Valmiki yelled at him not to talk that way. There was nothing he could do about it; he needed to support his family and his village who were in need and depended on him. They loved him and he could not fail them. He tied the *sadhu* to a tree and raised his sword to accommodate the *sadhu's* plea when the holy man exclaimed, "Wait! As a truthful being I must be fair to you and not leave this world in a half-truth. You should not kill me. I am a *sadhu*. If you kill me then you will certainly have the karma to die within a few days. Now you know. Please go ahead."

This perturbed Valmiki. He knew that saints' words always come true because the power of God lives in their tongues. He held back the fatal cut and asked, "I know what you say will come to pass. Is there no way to escape this destiny?" The saint replied, "If a member of your family will voluntarily die at the same time I do, die for you out of love, then you will be spared. But I do not think they love you that much."

Valmiki secured the saint to the tree and went to his village. He called together his entire clan and explained the situation. "I must kill this holy man to uphold my reputation. I cannot let it be known that someone escaped my hand. I have supported you all for years with my courage and my sword. Who now loves me enough to sacrifice for me?" No one moved forward to confirm his confidence in their love. He pleaded again and again. They started to yell at him and insult him. They said his actions were on his head alone and to ask them to sacrifice was insane. When he realized he could persuade no one, he returned to the holy man. He sat next to the saint and loosened his bonds. Valmiki became very depressed. His mind fogged over with memories of all he had done. He sensed the weight of all his karma and sins. He felt a deep confusion about life. He was never taught how to love, how to be loved, how to be spiritually great. Yet he had tried to act out of duty.

The saint saw his bewildered condition. He saw that ignorance surrounded the man but his soul had a sincere desire to understand the truth. The great saint had compassion. He touched the thief's forehead with his fingertips and with a blessing cleared the subconscious of its fears and ignorance. The thief looked up with clear eyes in blissful devotion. He said, "Great man, you have given me the vision of my true self; of my unlimited being—pure and without enmity. Give me some practice, some kind of sadhana, so I can master this consciousness and teach it to others."

The holy man gave Valmiki a kriya. He told Valmiki to chant "Ram" with no other thought in his mind and with no movement until the *sadhu* returned from his journey. Valmiki sat for many days without moving and went deep into the meditation. The same personality that gave him the discipline and alertness he needed to become a great *dacoit*, a master thief and head-cutter, was now his best ally to meditate with power and sincerity. When the *sadhu* returned several days later (some stories say it was years and that an anthill formed around him as he stayed motionless in absorption), he whispered the mantra in his ear and brought him out of his meditative trance. His sadhana had cleared away his tumultuous mind and all his karmas.

Valmiki, the highway *dacoit*, the highway killer and looter, became Rishi Valmiki. He reached a point of absorption in which he could write that which was to come. He wrote the *Ramayana* before the birth of Lord Ram! That is called "intuition." Through his sadhana, his intuition joined him with the Infinite; "*tat,*" the finite forms, joined with the "*sat,*" being beyond form. Man becomes God. That capacity is why you are told you are made in image of God. When you find that reality, you become that reality. And that is the beginning of real consciousness.

Compassion, as well as its partner forgiveness, comes with sadhana. Compassion and kindness are the highest virtues. As in the story of Valmiki, compassion can awaken and reshape the life of the lowest, grossest person into the highest, most refined person. It is important to realize that this happens not by detachment but by nonattachment. Nonattachment to your own ego lets you fully open the doors of the heart and the windows of perception. When you become still, zero in your ego, then compassion can flow through you. In that condition your connection with the universe and with others is changed. It seems like a miracle; but it is actually just a law that connects the formless infinity of creative being with this moment in which we face a specific action and respond from a particular form.

One way of explaining this is to think of compassion as creating a kind of vacuum—for the law of action and reaction has been transcended. Nature does not love a vacuum and neither does God. So s/he rushes to the service of that saint who acted with compassion. God must assist that consciousness for it is the expression of the highest, exalted form of God, Itself. There is a story about Guru Nanak, a great yogi and founder of the Sikh tradition, which shows this effect in action:

During the years when Guru Nanak lived a householder's life, he was in charge of a storehouse which issued grain to the Nawab's servants in Sultanpur. For three years he gave grain to all who asked for it, according to their need. A rumor came to the Nawab that Nanak was recklessly giving away grain and that the royal stores were now empty. The Nawab ordered an investigation. Very carefully the records were checked and the grain was weighed. Not only was the storehouse full of grain, but there was even more than was to be expected. The Nawab discovered that Nanak refused no one their needs and as Nanak counted out the measures of grain he would reach the number thirteen and begin to endlessly repeat the number, *tayra*, which also means "yours." He would say, "Yours, O God, I am yours," as he gave away all the grain. In a trance-like ecstasy, he was focused only on a state of merger with his Beloved and he always distributed more than was stored. Guru Nanak's service to the people in compassionately filling their needs created a "vacuum," an empty storehouse which was then filled by the One who gives everything.

In the stage of *prabhupati*, prosperity is assured. There is never a feeling of scarcity or a need to get something from someone else; because the Giver, that gives all, is giving to all. In this way, life becomes about actions that serve, create and express. There is no need to search for God or to get things from outside our Self. Instead the job of this stage is to recognize God in all and to act in oneness with that; you are engaged with each detail of life and every moment of the day is a realized sadhana. There is no moment when you are asleep or unaware of the present requirements of the universal consciousness. You cease to do what is right only for you and begin to do what is right for all.

For a practitioner of Kundalini Yoga, the experience of sadhana is a daily initiation. There is no need for any other initiation. No one in 3HO ever initiates anyone into a kriya or a secret mantra. There is no secret between us and God, so there should be no secret between us about God. The way to the infinite is clear. It is open to all. It may be clouded by our own ignorance, fears or lack of discipline, but it is already present in each of us. The real meaning of initiation is to make a confirmed beginning and let go of your limitations or ego. Every morning in sadhana, you bow before the Infinite. Your higher Self initiates your lower self and that is the secret of all secrets. The whole world assists you in this daily initiation.

As you begin sadhana, there is nothing around you except darkness. Worldly activity is at a minimum. As you sit and meditate on the infinite Creator, the day slowly dawns. Every cell of your being learns that meditating and chanting the *Nam* leads from darkness to light. The entire subconscious is alert to the primal experience of dawn and senses a renewal. The mind crystallizes, becomes sensitive and fills with trust of the higher Self's demands. When the mind is led past its ignorance and error to awareness, this is true initiation.

Anyone who practices a perfect sadhana begins to glow. They gain the ability to guide and inspire others. Just being in her or his presence helps clear your mind of useless conflicts.

Mental Structure

Each person has a mind that is unique. Its experience and understanding is formed from and limited by the structures and neural pathways generated from patterns of care during early childhood, surrounding culture, *samskaras* from past actions, the physical capacities of the body—neural, glandular and muscular, significant social relationships, nutritional history, physical and cognitive activities, and more. This rich matrix floods us with experience.

A major task in each moment of life is to integrate all that experience in a way that is meaningful and effective given the circumstances and intentions of the individual. The best catalyst for the individual mind to grow and integrate its experience is to experience merger in the universal mind. This immersion into the universal mind forms a relationship between your known and your unknown; creates stillness in the hyperactive, individual mind; and engenders choice and awareness. We develop our sense of self, our capacity for subjective experience and our ability for metacognition (ability to observe our own mind) through this relationship to the Infinite. Every experience the individual mind has of the universal mind contributes to the growth of a guiding consciousness. Every sadhana that embeds us into the sense of the Infinite, especially during the twilight hours when we are bound neither by the earth nor the heavens, builds that consciousness. With the expanded sense of self and the ability to let in the vastness of reality as it is, our aura also changes. It expands and refines. As it increases its sensory acuity, it gains in strength and stability. The result is that your presence—the space and connections of your auric body—becomes a catalyst; your presence works even when words cannot. People will feel uplifted and naturally guided just by being around you. The clarity and energy of your presence induces a similar clarity within them so that they can realize their own consciousness and intelligence. This is a quality of the Kundalini Yogi, of authentic teachers from any tradition, and certainly of a Kundalini Yoga teacher. We are all, at our core, teachers for each other.

Three Approaches to Consciousness

Pratyahar

In yoga there are three main approaches we use to connect the individual mind to the universal mind and build our consciousness: *pratyahar, laya* and *shuniya*. First we'll look at *pratyahar*. In this method, you inject the universal mind into the individual mind by a contraction and synchronization process. You open your mind widely to notice all the thoughts that flow

through it then process each thought pattern. If you do not "process" the thoughts, filter them through your consciousness, the thoughts will process you by shaping your actions, reactions and feelings through the mix of conscious, subconscious and unconscious impressions and patterns. Without the skill to process the flow of thoughts, we can be very robotic, habitual and reactive. We can lose our purpose under the pressure of circumstance or act from the habits of our ego instead of from the spontaneous creativity of our identity. When we successfully develop the discipline to process the flow of thoughts, we can deny a thought, create a thought, implant a thought, attract things with our thought and understand the reality and consequences of our thoughts.

Thoughts can come from many sources: your intentional projection, your body, your surroundings, and even from the greater galaxy itself. No matter where the thoughts arise from, we must process and qualify each thought through our consciousness. We must qualify a thought in that we accept it or reject it. Does the thought serve my consciousness? Are the consequences of the thought something that I wish to accept? Most the time we follow our thoughts. We chase them as if they are a reality.

The yogi has discovered that consciousness and the mind are two different things. The mind is largely automatic. Its constant flow of thoughts and feelings is largely not conscious. Consciousness comes from our being. To the yogi, consciousness is as primary as time, space and energy. It exists without form as well as within form. Consciousness, in this sense, is in addition to the thoughts rather than being composed by the thoughts. We can look without seeing. We can listen without hearing. Consciousness is a capacity beyond the five senses or the flow of thoughts; in fact, it can even exist without thought at all.

Normally we act and react off of the cues given to us by sensations that arise from feelings and thoughts, which makes us subject to the whims of our subconscious and the desires that arise automatically from the flow of thoughts. This is why certain emotions are pivotal to yoga practice. Compassion and forgiveness reduce the reactions to the thoughts that come from our negative or defensive mind. They quell the constant urges of the old brain to run, attack or withdraw. A yogi regains, respects and refines the self by letting go of all the thoughts. Nonattachment allows us to project a thought from our neutral mind and also step back from the perspectives created by the thoughts received from the positive or negative minds. These same constructive emotions are supported by the *yamas* and *niyamas*—the social and ethical imperatives—of Patanjali's eight-fold path of yoga practice.

The yogi cultivates subtlety and intuition residing within the neutral mind and beyond in intuitive awareness. The yogi learns to sense consciousness itself. From that awakened observer position, we can cultivate our sense of self, our consciousness and the power of our awareness. One of the primary functions of a good sadhana is to pass each thought through the filter of our consciousness.

The practice of *pratyahar* cultivates the clarity of the senses, the subtlety of perception and the crystallization of self-awareness. *Pratyahar* is sometimes translated as "sensory withdrawal and control." Yogi Bhajan used two phrases to describe *pratyahar*: substitution or "contraction and synchronization." Substitution means replacing a "negative" thought with a "positive" thought. To put this in context, the entire world of the senses and experience, which we call *prakirti*, is called "negative" in relationship to the manifold realm of existence that is universal and non-dual which is called "positive". This is a philosophical distinction fundamental to yoga cosmologies. Sometimes we refer to the spirit and the body, or the earth and the heavens. In this way, the two core processes of unity in the spirit and diversification in the body/mind are

expressed. To substitute a thought from the negative to positive means to sense the subtle aspects of thought and add a thought from the universal mind. To connect the negative or limited sense of a thought to consciousness is to go beyond thought and mind, to reset the individual mind, beset by attachments and particulars, toward a universal mind that admits the play of spirit, being and consciousness to manifest through mind into form.

Each thought comes cloaked in subconscious sensations, associations and desires. Through the intuitive mind, you can sense not just the qualities of the thought but the presence of the giver of the thought as well. You can sense the origin, context and karma of the thought, not just its trajectory. Through substitution, we remove the tentacles that enmesh the thought and prevent it from being seen clearly. Then we synchronize this clarified thought with consciousness itself. Instead of being entangled with the thought and all of its attendant emotion and commotion, we maintain clarity in our consciousness and see all the implications of the thought—past, present and future. "Contraction" is when we intentionally move from this vast universal consciousness to dwell on one thought. It is with our power of contraction that we can peel away the layers that surround the thought to understand its essence—it's *antar*. In *pratyahar*, we deal with thoughts as they are. We add to the thought the qualification of our consciousness. It's a powerful practice that releases the mental hypnosis induced by our thoughts, emotions, and commotions and puts consciousness on the throne of our actions.

Yogi Bhajan has elaborated in detail how the mind works, using the positive, negative and neutral minds within it. In his book with Gurucharan Singh Khalsa, *The Mind*, he explains how thoughts become cloaked and how the 81 facets of our mind function as subtle nuances in the play of projections. The most important process for sadhana is simply to provoke the subconscious to release its thoughts, so that your consciousness can synchronize the thought and transform it from gross to the subtle, from the negative to the positive and from the mind to the Being.

Laya

The second method is *laya*. The word itself means suspension and implies absorption, levitation or a devotional merger. *Laya* suspends the Self directly into a sense of the Infinite rather than finding the infinite within a thought or a finite object. You recognize nothing in yourself except the infinite; you admit no limitation. *Laya* techniques take you from the individual mind to the universal mind. You suspend the activities of the normal flow of thoughts and actions and focus instead on limitlessness, vastness and the totality of what exists. In the nature of your essential being there are no limitations. Limitations arise because we live in the world of *prakirti*, and the laws of polarity that govern this plane of existence. Laya Yoga always involves the use of mantra and rhythm, often with a special breathing pattern—the mind is absorbed through sound. We hear a mantra but at the same moment we hear the origin of the mantra in the unmanifest Being. Subtle sounds and *Naad* pervade every cell. The meridians in the body clear. The kundalini proceeds through the chakras increasingly refining and expanding the energy.

From this practice, the mind lets go of its outwardly directed activity. It becomes desireless and finds happiness, bliss even, within itself and in the soul's being. Eventually the mind is stilled and the absorption in the pulsations of the inner sound—the *Naad*—releases spiritual powers and enhanced mental abilities. Whatever a yogi dwells on in this state is similarly awakened or blessed. As we absorb our Self into the vastness and absoluteness of the Infinite and God, we dissolve all the difficulties, negativity and karma that beleaguer our path.

These techniques are often identified with the skillful use of and attention to the chakras and with special mantras unique to Kundalini Yoga. Yogi Bhajan recorded many of these mantras and techniques and took them from under the ancient cloak of secrecy and initiation and revealed them to us all so that they might serve us as we serve all in the Aquarian Age. The Laya Yoga form of the Adi Shakti Mantra is one of the most powerful of these legacies. Yogi Bhajan, in a parallel manner, contrasted *pranayam* to *pratyahar* as a technique that expands you into the vaster sense of the cosmos as it increases your energy and awakens each cell and meridian. In the philosophy of yoga, the universe, in its unmanifest state, is in *pralaya*, when all of the objects of creation are absorbed into Being itself, God's sleep. There is a cycle of creation that manifests all things: from the great *mahapralaya*—final suspension—into the activity of *prakirti* then back again to a condition of *laya*. Actually these processes go on together, as interdependent co-creating polarities, free from our linear sense of time. Non-existence and existence feed each other in the great, cosmic, dynamic dance.

Laya techniques use this never ceasing flow to release the blocks that arise from attachment, ego and the *tattvas*. They open the intuition and are a source of seemingly miraculous healing and prosperity. A Kundalini Yogi masters both *pratyahar* to control the mind and strengthen its projection, and *laya* to move diagonally between the polarities of life with intuition as a guide. These two approaches are the right and left hands of the contemplative mind of the yogi.

Shuniya

The third method is to cultivate the state of *shuniya*. *Shuniya* is a state of absolute stillness. Yogi Bhajan called it the zero state. It is like a vacuum in which there is thoughtlessness. You neither react nor non-react to any thought, feeling or circumstance. You consolidate yourself into a state that has no boundary. It is a state free of ego that dwells in complete openness. *Shuniya* is both a state and a practice. As the state of shuniya releases the grip of your thoughts, as the presence of your consciousness increases, and as your awareness is touched by grace, you bloom into a condition of consciousness called *turiya*. This is an awakened stage, sometimes called *samadhi*. You embrace everything and yet you are beyond any one thing. You are yourself and yet within everything. You are in a flow in which every effort is effortless.

Shuniya is the gateway to *turiya*, a perfect awareness and realization of the merger of your finite and infinite Self. If *pratyahar* and *laya* are the left and right hands of contemplative practice, *shuniya* is its heart. The key to *shuniya* is to simultaneously experience two opposite states and deny both equally, releasing the hypnotic grip of the polarities that hold us into our illusions and neuroses. If you want to exist, meditate on non-existence. If you want to attract everything, let everything go and empty yourself. The universe has to balance energy and psyche; *shuniya* is its fulcrum. This is hard for many people to understand because we busy ourselves constantly trying to get things. We rarely relax and allow the universe to bring it to us.

Here is how Yogi Bhajan guided us into a basic *shuniya* meditation:

"To meditate into shuniya *is a very powerful exercise. Now close your eyes and sit down. Just personify that you are sitting in a place which is a vacuum—shuniya—nothing. If a person does not meditate on nothingness, he will not get everything. That's a law of nature that nobody can change. It's a law of prosperity, too. This is a prosperity which shall come to you. Why? Because you at this time are calling on that nothingness which is holding everything. Please don't hold to any thought. Meditate. Close your eyes in a simple posture like a saint. Technically speaking, just know nothing.* Shuniya.

There's a very simple theory, "God in all." You are in all, all is in you, nothing. Just sit into nothingness. Any thought which comes to you, say no. Like that child who grows to be a boy or girl, there comes a period when they say no to everything, remember. You are no different than that tonight. Technically speaking put yourself into the realm of no. You may end up experiencing a million things. Go with no thought. Bypass it. Be Zero; meditate on zero or a full stop—like a little point. Shuniya means that.

The constant thinking of the intellect can be stopped by this. There's no excitement in this condition. It's just that you are non-existence: no thought, no existence, nothing. No fear, no security. Don't agree to shake hands with any thought; if anything touches you, just say no. You don't exist. Practice "I am not." You are not learning, I am not teaching. There's a class but there's no class. You call yourself civilized; no, you are wild. You call yourself wild; no, you are civilized. But neither are you civilized, nor are you wild. Say no to everything. That's what you are practicing. No duality; non-duality. No good and bad. No right and wrong. No existence, non-existence. Now go beyond even that. Eliminate the intellect and all its thinking." —Yogi Bhajan, March 21, 1993

A flawless sadhana will create a profound transformational experience by entwining all three of these methods like three tightly woven strands of a strong rope. There are moments you must confront the mind as you quell the intrusive thoughts, redirect the errant thoughts, reject the impulsive thoughts and synchronize the flow of thoughts. There are moments you leave behind your concerns and enter beyond yourself into the ecstasy of the sound current. The burden of self-concern is temporarily removed like an old heavy backpack. And there are moments of complete stillness in which you are the entire world *and* you are nothing, then destiny, intuition and prosperity support every step of your journey in this life.

Each kriya of Kundalini Yoga and each sadhana that Yogi Bhajan gave us mixes these elements as Beethoven combined the notes, harmonies and rhythms in his best musical compositions. There is an inner necessity, a natural law that guides the refined sensitivity of any Master. So it was with Yogi Bhajan, who was a Master of the transformational power of kundalini and awareness. The sadhanas he shared with us over the years satisfied the needs of the times he gave them and guided us through a timeless catalogue that revealed the inner potentials of our minds and souls.

Group Sadhana and the Expanded Self

Sadhana is a discipline that moves us toward cosmic consciousness and self-realization; it creates individual excellence and helps to fulfill the destiny and potential of our soul. It may seem like a solitary enterprise, rising each morning and practicing mindfulness, qualifying each of our actions and thoughts throughout the day, because it does call on our individual will and commitment. In reality, however, the individual effort is supported and expanded by the group in group sadhana. Thus our task extends beyond mastery of our own minds into the mastery of group consciousness. Yogi Bhajan reminded his students that the stages of practice led from individual consciousness through group consciousness to universal consciousness.

There is individual consciousness and from there, group consciousness and then we reach universal consciousness. The aim of man is to reach universal consciousness. The Teachings of Yogi Bhajan, p. 117

Group consciousness is an intermediate stage. It is what you pass through in the journey from individual consciousness to universal consciousness.
The Teachings of Yogi Bhajan, p. 176

Group consciousness is our ability to communicate and be sensitive to others; to extend our awareness

and understand our part in something greater. Practicing our social skills is an opportunity to learn to rise above our ego, which typically defends itself, its likes and dislikes by isolating from others, or by dominating or projecting negative or positive qualities on others. When we are aware and use our intuitive neutral mind, the vast resources and energy of the universe, the psyche and potential of the environment, and the perspectives beyond the narrow confines of our ego are invited in. If we cannot drop our reactions to a person, how do we expect to be authentically open to our own vastness and to God which is radically beyond the small domain of our ego?

The three best ways to develop group consciousness are group sadhana, living in community, or doing service or seva with others. This is one of the reasons for the long tradition of yogic aspirants living in an ashram community where disciplines were practiced together under the scrutiny and corrective guidance of a Teacher, a Master of the practice. An ashram is the center of a community of practitioners, a place where everyone gathers in the early morning hours to do sadhana together. Literally, it means "house of the teacher." Members of an ashram community have their own lives and livelihoods and they act as servants and teachers to the higher consciousness which is the Teacher. A strong group sadhana is essential for an ashram to serve its role. In an ashram community if everyone did only an individual practice, gradually and inexorably the power of unity and group consciousness would wane and individuals would drift toward the normal ego, conflict-based thinking.

When Yogi Bhajan began the 3HO family he encouraged teachers to live in the world as householders, avoid ascetic withdrawal and, when possible, develop communities with a shared practice. Communities that share self-discipline, values and consciousness are called a sangat. Participation in a sangat, sangum or gathering of the holy is a central tenet in the wisdom traditions. Such communities develop the humility and kindness that must accompany wisdom and strength on the path of awareness.

There are two other benefits to the group process. When you do group sadhana, you multiply the effect of all the individuals and you invite growth and healing in areas of the self you may not have discovered on your own. When you participate in a community that holds common values and a commitment to the teachings, you have many ways to serve and many avenues of feedback and correction to keep your ego in check.

The techniques of Kundalini Yoga stimulate the basic evolutionary force in the psyche. As the urge to grow increases, each person feels the expansion of his or her own energy or shakti. As this energy increases the effects manifest in awareness, the ability for self-control, the ability to influence people, the effective application of the will, and the power of the intuition and sensitivity to subtle energies. At times the experience of expansion and the fading away of old patterns and fears can lead to spiritual ego in which pride and certainty collude with the emotions and needs of the subconscious and the ego to create the very opposite of the aspirant's intention. An expanded awareness does not guarantee mastery of the ego. Yogi Bhajan constantly cautioned his teachers to recognize the signs of spiritual ego so that they could avoid it. He said that it was less curable than cancer. It eats away at your connection to others, your clarity, and leads you to insulate yourself from the guidance and feedback of others. The potential for spiritual ego is perhaps one reason Kundalini Yoga, and the art of Raj Yoga, came through the House of Guru Ram Das, the fourth teacher of the Sikh tradition and a master of Raj Yoga. He exemplified and inspires the ideals of self-sacrifice, service, universal tolerance, acceptance, and humility.

It is important for a practitioner of any discipline that awakens the potential of the Self not to become too involved in the play of the ego. If all the energy developed and released in sadhana focused through the ego structure, the psyche of the student could become imbalanced, exaggerated and filled with intermittent impulses, fantasies or attitudes of entitlement, ego-inflation or narcissism. These spiritual crises are uncommon when there is a steady sadhana, a strong group consciousness and openness to feedback from a sangat.

The ego can transform and give way to the presence of the self and to the flow of consciousness. The ego development of a yogi goes through five major steps. The lowest is that of egomania—everything is valueless unless it corresponds to the individual's desire. There is no sympathy or understanding for another person. Words and actions are by impulse, fear or need. The Self has little sway and other people are seen as instrumental, not real or valued in their own existence. Yoga is done to get what they need or avoid what they fear.

The second step is egotism. A person in this stage is not as relentless in his ego; he appears arrogant rather than maniacal. He is aware of other egos as well as his or her own but always chooses personal needs over others. There is more flexibility in the personality but most actions are still impulsive or habitual.

The third step is ego-centeredness. In this stage, the person consciously develops strengths and capacities to reflect, to recognize and value others, to project goals through time and beyond immediate challenges. Yet, emotions and impulsive actions still prevail in most choices even though there is an increased need for consistency and meaning. The ego is more developed, stronger and allows in more perspectives, though limited, about others and about the world as it is.

The fourth step is self-centeredness. In this stage, the person opens their Heart Center and the sense of Self becomes greater than the identification with ego. This is the first step where a stable sense of Self and a relationship to the Self's presence develops. With a new identity centering on the Self, the yogi can step back from the emotions and redirect them. It is a stage that cultivates compassion for the Self and for others; that perceives others as real as one's Self; that can increasingly redirect or stop actions arising from impulsive thoughts or feelings; that can act beyond pain or pleasure. Once this stage blossoms it is often mistaken for the final step. The yogi begins to transcend the most rigid and limiting aspects of the ego and realizes an identity that admits a sense of a larger Self. This is often a delightful vision of the Self, full of discovery, pleasure and excitement.

But the truly final step is selflessness. There is still an ego; but it is a healthy ego—strengthened, balanced and functional—that serves the true identity, rather than being the center of the identity. The ego has released its hold and an experiential merger with the Infinite and the realms of non-dual reality replaces it. This is often thought of mystically, but it is only mystical to the ego. It is a stage of mastery, first of the Self then of consciousness. The yogi is not bound by any finite form; instead she acts with compassion and kindness to all from a non-dual awareness that is beyond the normal polarities of the mind. New capacities are awakened that are a natural part of being fully human. In this final step there is a merger with the practical sense of infinity. The Infinite has become intimate and pervades all normal activities like a constant background glow. Emotion flows with renewed range and intensity but devotion directs and qualifies each emotion to serve the identity, Infinity. Such a selfless yogi can be a mindful observer of even the most passionately initiated actions to see clearly the effects of those actions before they are performed. Neutrality and equanimity are the rule. The stage of selflessness gives the ability to forgive the past and live in harmony with the cosmos. In this stage, service and unbounded openness to the community are effortless. It is no longer a goal to gain face and grace

for the self; instead the Yogi provides the opportunity, inspiration and guidance for others to experience that grace. Even if the yogi feels a normal depression, lifting others from their depressions lifts the yogi's. This final stage passes through the group consciousness that both tests and supports it. Individually it is very rare. That is why Yogi Bhajan bemoaned the sad fate of yogis who had to be isolated in caves or remote locations for lifetimes of meditation. The full realization only dawned as they became a part of everyone. This is what the Buddha showed clearly in the teachings of the Bodhisattva; what Christ exemplified in healing and accepting everyone regardless of status, tribe or belief; and what the Sikh Gurus demonstrated in removing the barrier between the Guru and the student and giving equal status to the Infinite that resides in us all.

By living in a community that shares the same teachings, lifestyle, and consciousness, it is very difficult to do some spurious action that opposes the new consciousness. Everyone, or at least someone, will notice and give you helpful feedback and encouragement to help you keep to the clarity of your dharma—the expression of your consciousness. As much as we like to change instantly, the subconscious mind and old patterns form at least 60% of our actions. A strong group can help you provoke, clear out and train that deep part of the mind. On your own, you might find the one clean room in the house and stay in its inviting atmosphere instead of doing the hard work of a thorough cleaning, making every space functional and inviting. In an ashram community, you become skilled in making decisions that incorporate the needs of the community; learning to listen and communicate harmoniously; balancing your personal agendas with the values and strategies of the groups and teams involved. This experience lays the foundation for acting as an enlightened leader and conscious community member with values engendered by an open heart and an applied consciousness.

Group sadhana develops a higher interpersonal sensitivity in such a community. At the beginning of a group morning sadhana, everyone has a different vibration. Some have traces of dreams, other's minds are already filled with concerns of the day, and still others come with a great variety of needs and expectations about the results of doing sadhana together. The more people there are, the more these individual differences balance and cancel each other out. The happiness of one person balances the sadness of another. The alertness of one person balances the sleepy drift of another. Gradually the entire group finds its energy directed by the activity of the sadhana itself. The individual auras merge and form a group aura. If the group is tuned in to the Infinite, a "rainbow aura" forms that reflects all colors and hovers over the group like a sacred signature of light written by their higher selves. A bluish color of clarity, calmness and devotion predominates. One hour of sharing this type of energy can erase the effects of a week of arguments and discord, massive amounts of stress and change, and add a window of opportunity to see clearly how to excel and succeed that day. The strength of a community is directly proportionate to the strength of their group sadhana. This auric transformation aids each individual practitioner to make the step beyond ego centeredness to selfless awakening.

By the end of morning sadhana, when everyone's energy has intermingled and merged, it is easy to communicate and be on the same wavelength. You see this effect throughout the day. There will be fewer misunderstandings in the area of communications. If your sadhana is done as a couple or a small group the sense of connection, communication and strength is equally profound.

If you are not in an ashram community, see if there is a local ashram or yoga center where you can practice. Treat your own home as an ashram in which you invoke your higher consciousness, practice sadhana

and where you open your doors to others. It is easy and rewarding to welcome a few friends, fellow yogis or members of your family to practice with you occasionally, daily or for special gatherings. We are not born alone; nor should we live alone. Gather together and experience your greatness in sadhana.

The Practical Structure of Sadhana

The essence of a good sadhana is constant practice. Nothing, absolutely nothing, replaces the value and effects of practice. Without it, all studies, writings, and hopes become empty and meaningless.

There are many kinds of sadhanas which we outline in the next essay. We will describe here some ideal structures for a complete universal sadhana that guarantees optimal results to the vast majority of participants.

Physical Environments

In meditatition, sadhana and deep prayer you become supersensitive. The environment that surrounds you has a huge effect on the ease of going into meditation and the ease of maintaining the depth of meditation. Colors, sounds, smells and even the past use of the room register in your consciousness and affect its energy and yours. Designing a beautiful, serene meditation room is an ancient art that is now in the mainstream culture, so there are many resources and guides to help you create your own sacred space. When it is done well, just entering the room or the space of a small altar automatically draws one into a meditative state just like the vastness of an ocean vista or the silence of a an old-growth forest.

The first step is to choose a place that is used primarily or entirely for sadhana. It should always be kept perfectly clean and neat so it reminds you of your clarity, devotion and most subtle consciousness. Create an aesthetically pleasing arrangement of pictures, plants and objects that have special meaning for you. The meditation room should smell fresh. Let air circulate and keep the temperature moderate, if possible. Too much cold may harm the body in deep meditations. Too much heat will induce sleep and poor circulation. Cover the spot you sit on with an animal skin or a wool blanket since they insulate your psycho-electromagnetic field from the electromagnetic field of the earth. If a skin or proper fabric is unavailable, the next best substance to sit on is wood. As you become calm through meditation, you become more sensitive to the waves of energy within and without. Before you began a meditation practice, you may have required a high level of constant change and stimulation to be alert. Now stimulation from the inner Self is enough. Sharp noises and constant interruptions should be minimized during meditation and sadhana. In intermediate stages of meditation the normal sound of a door closing may feel like an explosion. Of course, there are specific sadhana practices in which we choose to sit in noisy and disruptive environments to build steadiness and concentration under challenge. But for normal meditation it is best to cultivate our practice steadily and choose supportive environments. For a graceful meditation choose a graceful environment.

The Physical Self and the Wake Up Routine

Create a purification ritual that you never fail to perform. Wake yourself gently in the morning and do the standard wake-up exercises. Before you wake in the morning, your mind gives you a signal to awake. At that signal, turn on your back with your eyes closed. Make your hands like cups and place them over your eyes. Look into the palms and slowly raise your hands to 1 ½ feet. Do Cat Stretch several times to each side: One knee comes to the chest and across the body as the arm stretches up. Stretch Pose for 1-3 minutes with Long Deep Breath or Breath of Fire. Relax for 2-3 minutes. Then bring both knees into the chest to release gas. Rock back-and-forth to massage the spine. Sit up and come into Easy Pose with the arms straight

and the hands in Gyan Mudra on the knees. Take at least 26 long, deep, complete breaths. Feel energy charging the bloodstream and the breath recharging every cell in your body. Then, to build your aura, put your arms at 60° for Ego Buster (fingertips pulled in tightly to the pads of the hands) with Breath of Fire for 1-3 minutes. Inhale and bring your thumb tips together over your head. Then exhale and continue your wake up routine.

Remember to drink a few glasses of water. Take either a cold shower or do a sequence of cold-warm-cold showers. Traditionally as you shower and cleanse the body you clear the mind with positive thoughts, mantra or spiritual songs. Let the clear flow of the water clean your aura of nighttime thoughts. Stimulate your circulation to flush the residues of nocturnal cleansing out of your body. You cannot meditate easily if your circulation is still in patterns suited for sleep or drowsiness. Massage the whole body, especially the feet, hands, face and ears while in the shower. If you are extra kind to yourself rub almond oil on your skin before you get into the shower. This simple treatment will maintain the health of the skin and calm scattered thoughts and anxious feelings.

After your shower, wear clothes that are comfortable, loose, flexible, and neat and clean. White is the best color for sadhana clothes. This color reflects all colors and it automatically adds several inches to the aura. Do not wear the same clothes to sadhana that you wore to bed. You must communicate to your consciousness in any way you can that sadhana is a special activity. Conscious attention to how you dress will help your mind be more alert and far more cooperative because it knows an important event is about to take place.

Before starting the practice of *Japji* and Kundalini Yoga, cover the head with a natural fiber cloth. Ideally this is white cotton. In many traditions it is a turban or scarf. It modulates the smooth functioning of the seventh chakra and creates subtle protection over the flows of energy released in deep meditation. If you use a meditation blanket or shawl, choose a natural fiber—wool, silk, or cotton—and use it only for meditation. Over a period of time the shawl will gain the same qualities as the meditative space and anchor the attitudes of meditation. Eventually, just putting it on will aid your efforts.

Mental Environments

After the physical environments are prepared, set your mind for sadhana and toward group consciousness—the more people in the group the better. When you chant by yourself you are only one voice; by chanting with others, the effect of your sound is multiplied by the others and by their hearing and reflecting your voice. If you must do sadhana by yourself, then while you are chanting, visualize a million others all around you. Hear them all chanting; place yourself in the center. Become completely still. Even as you chant and meditate, feel as if it is not you who chants; but rather, the chant vibrates in every cell of your body and flows through you like a current of sound. You are leading this million, receiving and giving blessings. This attitude is called "ajappa jap" or repeating while not repeating—spontaneous chanting. It is a mental state of merger into the sound current. This is the secret of a good sadhana—you do not do sadhana, you are sadhana; you experience effortless effort and learn to act not from the ego but from the Self and consciousness. Suspend you regular mental patterns and place yourself in the hands of your consciousness; invoke, evoke and devote yourself to your higher Self.

If you lead group sadhana, pay attention and set the mental atmosphere for all participants by your own attentiveness, graciousness and presence. Take care of the logistics: check for unexpected visitors and guests and make them welcome and informed in how to participate, check the physical environments and be prepared to guide the sadhana exercises smoothly. Make any explanations brief so participants focus on the ex-

perience and not on you. Prepare your mind to project your words and tones from a positive mind, open and creative. With this mental attitude, you will have the altitude that gives you victory all day.

Mental Self

The most important step is to align your mind to the higher Self so your consciousness presides in the sadhana. Your higher consciousness is represented by the teacher. In Kundalini Yoga we link to that consciousness and energy through the Golden Chain by tuning in with three repetitions of the Adi Mantra: *Ong Namo Guru Dev Namo*, which means, I bow to the subtle divine wisdom, the divine teacher within. This consciously puts the ego asideand guarantees protection through the subtle body of the teacher and Guru; it invokes an inflow of energy and light to your body and mind. It is an essential step in doing Kundalini Yoga. Meditate on your higher Self and your teachers, on Yogi Bhajan and Guru Ram Das as guides in that Golden Chain and feel that in all devotion and humility you are asking for guidance in sadhana. Pray that no matter how feeble your effort may be, the maximum benefit will be returned to help you serve humanity in the will of the Creator. Realize at this point that during sadhana the only teacher is the higher Self, the Guru, the flow of the teachings. Awaken yourself consciously to the fact that you do not know what the results of your efforts will be and dedicate the results to the infinite. This is the attitude of Karma Yoga exemplified in the *Bhagavad Gita* which asks us to be conscious of each act and to realize that there is always much more than our ego and focus are aware of. So in sadhana let the full results, much greater than you may imagine, be guided by the Infinite and the subtle soul of each person.

Sadhana brings energy and vitality to your mind and to your life. It also stirs up the subconscious, which sometimes looks like boredom, sleepiness and distraction. Even students who establish a strong regular sadhana can encounter a moment of boredom. Do not fight this; simply become more aware and present to the experience of it and soon enough it will shift on its own. Assess whether you have expectations that interfere with simply doing the sadhana. Many people seek a grand experience, a confirming miracle or relief from painful thoughts and feelings when in fact sadhana may temporarily intensify thoughts and feelings—comfortable or uncomfortable.

Instead, let your immersion into the vastness of the higher Self, the infinite sense of consciousness determine the experience of sadhana. Be present and aware, and allow all conflicts and tension to relax. Do not fight the mind, transcend it; do not seek something miraculous, recognize the miracle that is right now; do not look for control, delight in the control of the self within the flow of life and your mind.

When the mind engages sadhana in this manner, each moment is new. Just as the body constantly changes and renews, the mind increases its sensitivity and finds no place for boredom, only an experience of the uniqueness and power in each moment. Let your individual mind rest in the neutrality of the infinite mind.

The Essential Practice

Tune In

Always tune in with the Adi Shakti Mantra 3-5 times before beginning any Kundalini Yoga practice or meditation. After the whole group has tuned in, there are six important parts to the core of sadhana.

Physical Preparation

This physical body is the temple of God. It allows us to manifest consciousness and move about on the material plane. It must be exercised to keep the circulation balanced and strong, to remove tensions and blocks created by emotions, to alter the glandular secretions so they correspond to the state of consciousness you

want to attain, and to clean the blood system to prevent disease. Even with the best intentions and good thoughts, it is difficult to do a sadhana when you are sick. Take care of this physical body each day.

A strong exercise series awakens your will. You must push through minor aches and pains in order to have the strength and flexibility of both the muscles and the nerves that you need in order to face the day. This inflow of will power helps you beam the mind and stay alert during meditation and chanting. The exercises you practice should be sets as taught by Yogi Bhajan. They should leave you with a feeling of greater energy flow, an alert calmness, and enthusiasm. Too much exercise can tax the body so much that you will feel drowsy and lack motivation. A very heavy exercise and cleansing sadhana should be done when there is plenty of time to relax afterwards. A balanced series of exercises that works on breathing, nerves, glands and spine is perfect for sadhana.

Mantra

In every morning sadhana, we explore the power of mantra. Physical effort alone does not complete the subtle sublimation of the mind. Sadhana's affect rests on the fulcrum of some combination of these three elements: the basic kundalini mantra–the Adi Shakti mantra, an ashtang bij mantra and the Panj Shabd–Sa Ta Na Ma.

Guru Nanak said:

When the hands and body
are covered with dirt,
Water can rinse them clean.
When the clothes are dirty
and smeared with soil,
Soap can remove the stain.
When the mind is polluted
by error and shame,
It can only be cleansed by
the love of the Name.

The *Nam* is the main solvent for mental stains. This is very sensible. The breath rhythm gives you access to the subconscious as well as the conscious mind. When you chant these mantras, your mind is fixed on the infinite aspects of yourself. You do not relate to polarities. You go into the neutral mind in order to successfully clean out the fears and patterns in the subconscious. If a negative thought or fear comes to you, let it come, but be conscious of the rhythm of *Sa Ta Na Ma* or *Sat Nam*. With this *bij* mantra, the thought does not receive its standard resistance or reaction it usually gets when coming into consciousness, so it moves more into the center of your consciousness to provoke a reaction. The fear or thought lives on the energy you feed it by either positive or negative attention. By focusing on the infinite you appear neutral even if you become temporarily emotional. Because you are neutral, no reaction is returned to the thought or subconscious fear and it becomes neutralized. If you choose instead to fight the thought, you merely give it energy by giving it identity. With the mantra, you confirm your identity as the infinite truth and universal existence. Your mind may object, so let yourself ride on the mantra beyond the mind. If you decide to love the thought and become entranced by it, you will still give it identity. So to stop the continual production and maintenance of the dualities of consciousness, you must become neutral. This is ultimately achieved only through mantra, because sound is the basic creative potential of your being.

While there are many mantras Yogi Bhajan taught that can be practiced as a part of your daily spiritual practices, we have a basic morning sadhana which Yogi Bhajan gave in 1992, to be practiced until the year 2012. It is called the Aquarian Sadhana and consists of seven parts; it is described on pages 57-8. We also provide an entire history of the sadhanas Yogi Bhajan gave over the years to provide perspective on the development of the Aquarian Sadhana and an overall view of the various forms of 2½ hour practices.

Meditation

Doing mantra is a meditation. Any activity done in the right state of mind is a type of meditation, but here the reference is to silent meditation. It is that point in sadhana where you plunge into the total depths of the self with no outward stimulation to maintain you. This is where you test how well your inner being has awakened to support you. After every chant, take a few minutes to sit completely still without any movement and try to listen to the cosmic echo of the sounds you just produced. They are all around you, vibrating in the ether. If you can catch the subtle sound it will carry you without effort beyond the body consciousness into the sublime realms of self and bliss. It is for this that Guru Nanak said:

By the hearing of God's Name
Even the blind find their way.
By the hearing of God's Name
One grasps the infinite.
O Nanak, the Devotee is
Ever in bliss:
By hearing the Lord's Name,
His pain and sin are destroyed.

After every exercise you should rest a minute and meditate to integrate the changes, experiences and sensitivity the exercise created. By practicing meditation after a kriya, you will be able to regain the state of consciousness produced by that kriya any time during the rest of the day by a few seconds of meditation.

Deep Relaxation

After exercises, chanting and meditation, you should deeply relax. The ability to relax is a divine quality. You are more centered within yourself and you become more sensitive to the energy patterns of your life. The effects of the kriyas and chanting are cumulative. They build for a long time after you have done them. Allow time for the energies you have released in the body and mind to circulate and come to equilibrium without involving your ego as the "director of the show." The energy knows where it should go; it is automatic. During relaxation you should cover your body with the meditation blanket or shawl so that you do not get cold. The amount of time you spend in deep relaxation depends on what you have done. Normally you should rest between 10 and 20 minutes. The state of consciousness you experience in this deep relaxation will not be just sleep. The glandular balance in the blood is altered, as is the functioning of the brain. You may have out-of-body experiences, you may have vivid dreams, you may remember nothing at all after closing your eyes. You will not, however, go into a regular shallow sleep unless you continue relaxing for an extended time. The best position for deep relaxation is corpse pose: lie on your back with your arms at the sides, palms up, ankles uncrossed and eyes closed.

Kirtan

After you journey through inner space, you must always reconnect with the world and daily duties. Sit with everyone and have a fun sing along, singing the praises of the Infinite and the joys of life. Kirtan is an active singing rather than a deep meditation. It is the harmony of voices and instruments. It is realizing you are in a group of people who have purified themselves and are ready to actively live the day in truth and righteousness. Kirtan lets you re-enter worldly consciousness but with a difference. You tend to remember the tunes throughout the day and with every breath, utter the *Nam*.

Prayer

Prayer is a potent capacity in man. Prayer is when the finite consciousness addresses the infinite Self. Open your heart and be thankful for all the people who created and carried this consciousness through time so you could enjoy it now. You can ask for anything you want in prayer, for the Giver is infinite, and He gives

all. If one's heart can open in compassionate prayer for humility, every heartbeat can bring a miracle.

In the Sikh tradition, we always offer the Ardas which reminds us of our historical predecessors and our present duty to uphold consciousness and righteousness. A very universal way to offer a prayer is to dedicate part of your life force to what you pray for. Yogi Bhajan often gives an example of a prayer such as the following, which uses the breath:

Inhale and hold your breath,
For the peace of the world,
For the health of all, to make everybody happy, So those who are lonely may have their partner, And God may find mercy on everybody, on each individual.
Say this prayer on this breath
And please exhale.
This is the charity of the breath.
Inhale again.
Pray for all dear ones, related ones, known, unknown, on the whole planet, for those who are sick, those who are unhappy, unhealthy or need spirit.
Send this thought by doing a prayer on this breath, let it go.
Inhale deep again to end all causes and effects which affect any man and make him unhappy, for anything that brings war and destruction, for anything which brings hatred and jealousy.
Say a prayer on this breath
and let it go.

The universality of prayer for self-guidance and humility is shown in this prayer given by Yogi Bhajan at the end of a class:

Oh Formless in every form,
Oh Infinite of every finite,
Oh Unknown, known through the entire creation,
Oh, Beyond, still bound by love,
It was Thy grace that you spoke and You heard,

You made it possible that all people, Thy creatures,
could come and could share Thy grace.
Give us power to walk on the path of righteousness;
Give us humility to serve and find love of our brother;
Give us tranquility and peace to find the
higher realms of consciousness.
May Thy grace lead us to the light of infinity;
May our trip to the world be successful to spread
Thy service so the fellow mankind can share.
May this day bring us a peaceful onward journey.
May Thy grace prevail,
And may You lift us to the levitated consciousness.
Oh God of Gods,
Oh Lord of Lords,
if you have been so kind and merciful to bring us
together with Thee,
Oh Infinite, oh Unknown, oh Beyond
Still bound by love.
Give us the power of happiness, joy and bliss,
so we can live in the ecstasy of consciousness.
Sat Nam.

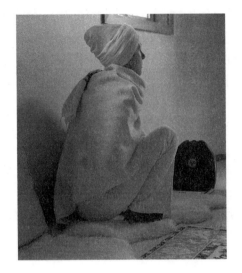

Models of Sadhana

A Complete History of Sadhanas Given by the Master
by Gurucharan Singh Khalsa, Ph.D.

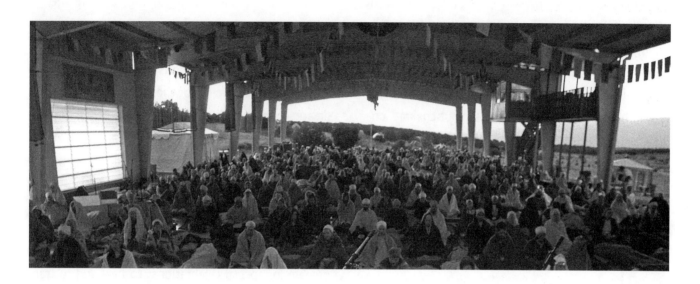

It seems that on a daily basis, when you do sadhana, nothing happens. But you don't do it out of greed. You do it to conquer your laziness, your ego, your stupidity, with your essence of commitment. That's all sadhana is. We don't do it to get anything.

—*Yogi Bhajan*

When this brief sadhana guideline was first put together, it was at the beginning of Yogi Bhajan's mission to share Kundalini Yoga and the technology for a happy, holy way of life. We now revisit these guidelines after practicing many sadhanas that he gave over the years and experiencing their structure. We have the benefit of hindsight and experience and now present a comprehensive overview of his collection of teachings.

Yogi Bhajan gave us the core of a great sadhana and many ways to begin implementing a personal practice. He gave us an ideal practice and then encour-

aged us to do something every day—no matter how small—that would gradually advance us toward the entire morning discipline as he outlined it; in turn we would receive the gifts of sadhana: a consciousness that extends throughout the day in all of our activities and a grace that covers all of our efforts.

In the same spirit as the original manual, we will present several models for a good sadhana and some suggestions on how to develop your own practice. We begin with a brief perspective and historical synopsis.

The First Sadhana

Yogi Bhajan started teaching by sharing the mantra that would stir the kundalini energy, balance the chakras and awaken the dormant consciousness and intuition in each of us. Without secrecy or initiation he gave, to anyone who would practice, the secret of the ages: *Ek Ong Kar, Sat Nam Siri, Wahe Guru,* also known

■49

as Morning Call or the Adi Shakti Mantra and translates as, "The Creator and all creation are one. This is our True Identity. The ecstasy of this wisdom is great beyond words." He tested this mantra himself and handed it out on a single sheet of paper with instructions to chant it for 2½ hours before sunrise, in what are known as the ambrosial hours. This was the first requirement of a student studying to become a teacher of Kundalini Yoga. It was the core practice, because it rapidly confronted the ego and took the practitioner through extraordinary states to the still clarity of awareness itself. This mantra was technical—about chakras, energy and subtle sounds; it integrated all the senses—body and mind; it was spiritual—pure and universal. Awareness was its core, its central technique and its result. He declared, at that time, that Kundalini Yoga was first and foremost about awareness; hence it became known as the Yoga of Awareness.

The practice of this mantra was the core sadhana for the first few years. Done in its long form, it opened all the chakras. The sound itself guided its flow through the subtle centers. The breath commanded the nerves and nerve plexuses. This mantra tames the mind and clears the subconscious. Through it, we experience the oneness and unity of all things in God and consciousness; we awaken to the reality of our higher Self and open to the ecstasy of the vastness of God and Being. All this because of a simple, direct sadhana. It was as if we had lived in a grand house for many years with the windows locked and shuttered. This simple mantra opened all the windows and let in the light.

This practice was historically significant because it initiated the kundalini energy in each person at the beginning of their path and marked the beginning of his teaching in the West. There was a synchronicity in this that foreshadowed the profound effect it would have on us as individuals and the legacy of the teachings. During this period, he said that the kundalini energy would awaken globally and usher in a new awareness of what it means to be a human being in the Aquarian Age. He explained that it would start on the west coast of the United States and travel around the globe until 2012, when it would complete its course. Along the way, it would catalyze the overturn of old structures and ways of interacting; ossified religious practices, empty of spirit would be replaced with an exponential explosion of technology and knowledge, and a desire in the human heart to express their creative spirit and relate to their soul without the constraints that defined religions in the past. This sadhana was to prepare us for the coming Age, giving us greater mental stamina, physical endurance and the caliber that comes with character so that we could excel and serve as teachers during this grand transition and into the millenniums that follow. It remains a core sadhana and central practice for Kundalini Yogis.

We use the incredible power of this meditation to prepare for special celebrations, to heal and to transition into a profound prayerful attitude. Yogi Bhajan would often have us chant for 24 hours at a time in one or two hour shifts—passing the chant from person to person or group to group. We experienced and learned the science of the "sound current." The mind would find equanimity as the inner chatter gave way to the sonorous rhythms of the chant. The repetition of the mantra changed our metabolism and opened the nervous system to new levels of integration and capacity. He explained that it adjusted our impulses and awakened the higher glands of the hypothalamus, pituitary and pineal. He encouraged each person to test the techniques and not accept anything without experiencing it themselves. He gave us the language of the ancient scriptures, conveyed the technology faithfully and spoke of the future when all these techniques would be documented in an entirely new scientific language. As we practiced this first sadhana and grew as communities of healthy, happy and holy people, we celebrated our awakening by founding 3HO and KRI to share and record the authenticity of the teachings.

Even as more sadhana practices were added and explained over the years, the 2½ hour Morning Call remained a central experience. Individuals or groups would set aside time to practice it for 40 days. This sadhana turned on the power—once on, you could organize and elevate your inner life, illuminating each nook and cranny with other kriyas and practices.

Integrating the Song of the Soul—Japji Sahib

In 1978, Yogi Bhajan changed the routine. The foundation well-laid, he began to build the house. When we practice sadhana in the early hours, it is twilight—neither deep night nor day. In that neutral territory we cultivate a direct conversation with our soul, our higher Self and with consciousness itself. We learn to be and not to be at the same time. We confront the mind with *pratyahar,* entrance the soul with *laya,* and as we dwell in *shuniya,* we create a seamless identity with the Infinite.

He had us begin to recite—not read—but recite consciously, exactly, as mantra, *Japji,* a poem in *Naad* written by Guru Nanak. We would do it in a call and answer form—alternately reading the couplets by women and men (with the women beginning)—so we could both listen and recite as we learned. Alternating the voices coordinated the polarities within us around the still point of consciousness. This practice also united the consciousness of the group to enhance our projection. *Japji* uses sound to stimulate and balance all eight chakras, five *tattvas* and the three *gunas.* It balances the mind even as it confronts it with inspiring, elevated streams of thought, traversing the nature of awareness, spirit, the universe and life. Some people wondered if reading *Japji* was a religious act, because practitioners of the Sikh path recite this in the morning as well. He explained it in terms of his being a "spiritual scientist," one who used well-tested discoveries that were the legacy of our birthright

as humans, regardless of race, creed, or religion. As awareness increases, it is natural to engage the conversation of the soul and by doing so, clear the mind, crystallize the will and open the heart.

After *Japji* we would do a set of Kundalini Yoga and then 15 minutes each of these four mantras. He had us use specific postures and mudras with several of the mantras. All the mantras were chanted in a steady rhythmical way:

1. Adi Shakti Mantra or Morning Call:
Ek Ong Kaar, Sat Naam Siree, Wha-hay Guroo

> The Creator and all creation are one. This is our True Identity. The ecstasy of this wisdom is great beyond words.

2. Aad Such, Jugaad Such, Haibhay Such, Nanak Hosee Bhay Such.

> True in the beginning, True throughout the ages, True at this moment, Nanak says this Truth shall ever be.

> This was done sitting on the heels in vajrasana; the arms extended to the sides, upper arms parallel to the ground, bend the elbows so the forearms are perpendicular to the ground and the palms face forward. The fingers and thumbs are straight up and together. The hands are stiff as if pressing against something. The eyes are 1/10th open. The mantra is chanted four times on each breath in a rapid monotone.

3. Guru Gaitri Mantra:
Gobinday, Mukanday, Udaaray, Apaaray, Hareeung, Kareeung, Nirnaamay, Akaamay.

> Sustaining, Liberating, Enlightening, Infinite, Destroying, Creating, Nameless, Desireless.

> Sit in Easy Pose, eyes 1/10th open. Cross the arms over the chest with the right hand resting on the left

forearm near the elbow, and the left hand resting on the right forearm. Chant the mantra four times on a breath in a smooth, rhythmical monotone.

4. *Guru Guru Wahe Guru Guru Ram Das Guru.*

Wise, wise is the one who serves Infinity

This was done in Easy Pose using the original melody or with simple variations that preserved the Naad and rhythm, using the instruments and musicians available.

This is a classical flow: First, awaken the energy. In every sadhana, throughout the years, he used this mantra first. Second, let the creative spirit of the self express and move past blocks in the Self. Third, clear the blocks in the world, your karma and enemies who oppose you. Finally, connect to the healing realms of Guru Ram Das, who like a miracle touches your soul—through the neutral mind—with compassion and love. It is a beautiful, balanced way to begin the day and clear your way.

At this point he also introduced gurdwara, as done in the Sikh tradition. The function of the gurdwara was to instill the practice of listening to your higher consciousness via the command or "hukam" of the Guru's consciousness, which expresses the heart beyond mind and emotions. The *shabds* of the Siri Guru Granth Sahib are spoken from an awakened soul by the saints and Yogis of that tradition; this consciousness confronts the mind with the soul.

Yogi Bhajan also encouraged sharing a bit of food prepared with prayerfulness. At Guru Ram Das Ashram in Los Angeles, where he taught for many years, they served delicious mint teas and five or more blanched almonds and sometimes a traditional *prasad*, a delicious combination of wheat, butter and light sweetener.

Prosperity and Expansion

In 1980 he gave a sadhana that kept these four mantras in their original order but instead of including the asanas and mudras, he had us sit in a normal meditative posture (Easy Pose) with the eyes fixed at the brow point or held 1/10th open. Each mantra was practiced for 11 minutes each—the time it takes the nervous system to shift and consolidate the projection of mastery. In the tradition of numerology it represents the higher Self and the Teacher. He also allowed us to vary the musical arrangements of the mantras as long as the melodies preserved the core pulse of each mantra. It was as if we had learned to sense the core of both the energy and the *Naad* and could now hold it at the center of the meditation even as we created more and more musical variations, inviting the play of the *tattvas* to flow. After these four mantras he added one more for an additional 11 minutes:

Har Har Har Har Har Har Haree.
Creative Infinity in action

This mantra was done sitting in Virasana, on the right heel with the left foot flat on the ground close to the body and the left knee close to the chest. Virasana is known as Hero Pose or Warrior Pose; it is a position of courage. (You'll note that with this mantra, Virasana is done on the right side rather than the left.) The eyes are 1/10th open and the arms are crossed so the hands gently grasp and rest on the biceps. The arms are parallel to the ground. The chant is continuous with one beat between mantra cycles.

This mantra is an *ashtang* or eight-beat mantra—central to Kundalini mantras. It brings prosperity and creativity into every aspect of your life. Following the other chants, it brings a natural flow of manifestation from your intentions, beyond any personal struggle and notion of ambition into the prosperous currents of opportunity constantly given to you by the infinite.

During this period he reminded us to listen to the "echo" or "resound" of the mantra after we completed each chant. Sit still for about a minute and dwell in the pulse of the energy the mantra creates and expresses. All things have a sound; he asked us to listen to the echo of the mantra as if it came from the entire universe not just your tongue. This consolidated our constant practice of *sunni-ai*—deep listening.

Guidance and Protection to Fulfill Your Path

In 1981 he asked us to focus the eyes on the tip of the nose—the lotus drishti—in each meditation. He had us chant Wahe Guru, one of the two *bij* mantras of Kundalini Yoga and added a new mantra: *Ardas Bhaee, Amar Das Guru, Amar Das Guru, Ardas Bhaee, Ram Das Guru, Ram Das Guru, Ram Das Guru, Suchee Sahee*. This extraordinary mantra is a source of hope and brings to you all resources to fulfill your path. As we live a Spirit filled life, we are tempted by many things, both from within and without. As a natural part of spiritual growth, we have to face our own shadow, our doubts and illusions. This point of transformation and challenge on the spiritual path is known as *shakti pad* and can be a time of great growth. From this challenge, we are given the opportunity to choose: Do we follow our dharma or our karmas? Do we experience victory or tragedy? This mantra assures guidance and protection as we cross this precarious territory in our spiritual path. It protects you from your own folly and from becoming a victim of others'. It combines the energy of Guru Amar Das and the energy of Guru Ram Das and guarantees clarity and guidance—to sense the truth of your heart and to go past any temptation or diversion from the fulfillment of your soul.

During the mid-80s, Yogi Bhajan guided his students and businesses through challenges that were personal, national and international. This sadhana gave us the strength of our aura, clarity of our will and the power of our projection go through such challenging times with both grace and prosperity. Chant each mantra 11 minutes.

1. Adi Shakti Mantra:
Ek Ong Kaar, Sat Naam Siree, Wha-hay Guroo

2. Wahe Guru, Wahe Guru, Wahe Guru, Wahe Guru-Wahe Guru, Wahe Guru, Wahe Guru, Wahe Guru Wahe Guru, Wahe Guru, Wahe Guru, Wahe Guru Wahe Guru, Wahe Guru, Wahe Guru, Wahe Guru

I am in ecstasy when I experience the Indescribable Wisdom.

Sit in easy pose or in a natural meditative posture. Focus your eyes at tip of nose. Place both hands into a Prayer Pose at the center of the chest. Chant Wahe Guru 16 times in a steady rhythmical monotone, or you may add music.

3. Ardas Bhaee:
Ardaas Bhayee, Amar Daas Guru, Amar Daas Guru, Ardaas Bhayee, Raam Daas Guroo, Raam Daas Guroo, Raam Daas Guroo, Sachee Sahee

Ardas Bhaee is a prayer through mantra. If you sing it, your mind, body and soul automatically combine and, without having to say what you want, the need of life is adjusted.

Sit in a Easy Pose. Extend the arms in front of you at shoulder level. Bend the elbows and rest the right forearm of top of the left. The left forearm is underneath the right. The palms of both hands face down and the fingers are extended straight. The wrists are also straight. Focus on the tip of the nose. Chant or sing the mantra.

4. Wahe Guru – Wha-hay Guroo

I am in ecstasy when I experience the Indescribable Wisdom.

53

Sit in Virasan: sit on the left heel with the right foot flat on the floor and the right knee bent up close to the chest. Place both hands in Prayer Pose at the center of the chest. Once again focus the eyes on the tip of the nose. Meditate on the mantra: *Wahe Guru*. You can repeat the mantra one time on a breath or many times on one breath. Choose a number of repetitions and a rhythm and continue that practice for the entire 11 minutes.

5. Har Har Har Har Har Har Haree

For this meditation use Virasan but sit on the right heel—the opposite of the last exercise. Sit on the right heel, with the left foot flat on the ground and the left knee bent up near the chest. The arms are crossed with the hands grasping the biceps gently. Elbows are up so that the forearms are parallel to the ground. Eyes focus at the tip of the nose.

This sadhana awakens your awareness with the Kundalini mantra. Your projection is strengthened by both your heart and your throat centers using the 16-beat mantra. Your prayer is strengthened and your guidance is assured by the third mantra. Finally, you meditate into the ultimate infinity. You dwell in the bliss of the Creator. This sadhana enables you to act with courage and strength, consciousness and creativity. Your journey is begun and you are certain to reach the end you desire.

Balance, Protection and Prosperity through All Challenges

In 1985 he introduced a new sadhana. He told us to practice it for five years—until 1990. It was a time when he faced many challenges and believed it was possible he would suffer an early death. So he said this was to be our ongoing sadhana if he did not survive to give us another. Fortunately, he did survive this period and continued to provide a prodigious flow of teachings and guidance until 2004.

In this sadhana we practiced six mantras. Morning Call is there, of course, but now it is fourth in the sequence: Chant each mantra 11 minutes.

1. So that generations would live in peace:

*Aad Guray Nameh, Jugaad Guray Nameh,
Sat Guray Nameh, Siree Guroo Dayv-ay Nameh.*

I bow to the primal wisdom. I bow to the wisdom true through the ages. I bow to the true wisdom. I bow to the great unseen wisdom.

2. Beyond Shakti Pad with Ardas Bhaee, a guarantee of synchronization in your prayer.

Ardaas Bhayee, Amar Daas Guru, Amar Daas Guru, Ardaas Bhayee, Raam Daas Guroo, Raam Daas Guroo, Raam Daas Guroo, Sachee Sahee

3. Mantra for protection:

Aap Sahaaee Hoaa, Sachay Daa Sachay Dhoaa Har Har Har.

The Lord Himself has become my protector. The Truest of the True has taken care of me. God. God. God.

4. Morning Call to awaken the kundalini:

Ek Ong Kaar, Sat Naam Siree, Wha-hay Guroo

5. For Prosperity:
This mantra contains the eight facets of Self [See Guru Gaitri Mantra]. *Har* is the original force of Creativity. The four repetitions of *Har* give power to all aspects and provide the power to break down the barriers of the past:

Har Har Har Har Gobinday
Har Har Har Har Mukanday
Har Har Har Har Udhaaray
Har Har Har Har Apaaray
Har Har Har Har Hareeung
Har Har Har Har Kareeung
Har Har Har Har Nirnaamay
Har Har Har Har Akaamay

6. Mul Mantra to master the 108 elements and dwell in Raj Yoga, the royal, regal being:

Ek Ong Kaar
Sat Naam
Kartaa Purakh
Nirbho Nirvair
Akaal Moort
Ajoonee, Saibhang
Gurprasaad. Jap.
Aad Such, Jugad Such, Haibhee Such,
Naanak Hosee Bhee Such

The Creator and all creation are One.
This is our True Identity.
The Doer of everything.
Beyond fear.
Beyond revenge.
Image of the Infinite.
Unborn, Self-illumined.
This is the Guru's Gift. Meditate.
Primal Truth, True through all time,
True at this instant,
O Nanak, forever true

For this sadhana, he did not specify any particular mudras or postures. After 16 years of training and teaching, he left the music up to the teachers and musicians and our own sensitivity. The sequence of mantras begins with an invocation of all knowledge to bring us its guidance but also to provide a special peace within the heart. He said practicing this would allow generations to live in peace with each other. The second takes us past personal challenges and guarantees the power and acceptance of our prayers within our own soul. The third mantra grants protection and prosperity and has us rely on the Infinite to support us, rather than our own individual, limited efforts. The Kundalini mantra is followed by a mantra of total balance and prosperity. The sequence ends with a recitation of the Mul Mantra to give our consciousness absolute balance and royalty.

Grace, Fulfillment and Growth

In 1990, Yogi Bhajan added two more mantras and adjusted the sadhana for this period of growth. One of the new mantras, **Waah Yantee, Kar Yantee** came from the time of Patanjali , one of the earliest known teachers of the system of yoga. It invokes the power of the balance of the three *gunas* as we chant and meditate on the sound *Wahe Guru*. It tells our mind that in the play of the polarity of the universe, there is truly nothing but the infinite consciousness from which everything arises. It has the power of purity and is the mantra of the Khalsa—those who choose to live purely with grace and strength before their consciousness. The second new mantra is "*Rakhay rakhanahaar*". This mantra is taken from the last stanza of *Rehiras Sahib*—a traditional prayer of the Sikhs done as an evening meditation. He said that this mantra "is for protection against all negative forces, both inner and outer, which move against one's walk on the path of destiny. It cuts like a sword through every opposing vibration, thought, word and action."

The Adi Shakti mantra is chanted in the long form—or Morning Call. The rest are done with any appropriate musical pattern that preserves the *Naad* of the mantras. You can sit in any meditative pose. There is no specific eye focus. Chant each mantra 11 minutes.

1. Morning Call:
Ek Ong Kaar, Sat Naam Siree, Wha-hay Guroo

2. Waah Yantee, Kar Yantee, Jagat Utpatee,
Aadak It Whaa-haa, Brahmaaday Trayshaa Guroo
It Wha-hay Guroo
Great Macroself, Creative Self. All that is creative through time, all that is the Great One. Three aspects of God: Brahma, Vishnu, Mahesh. That is Wahe Guru.

3. Mul Mantra:
Ek Ong Kaar, Sat Naam, Kartaa Purakh, Nirbho Nir-
vair, Akaal Moort, Ajoonee Saibhang, Gurprasaad.
Jap. Aad Such Jugad Such Haibhee Such
Naanak Hosee Bhee Such

4. Aad Guray Nameh, Jugaad Guray Nameh,
Sat Guray Nameh, Siree Guroo Dayv-ay Nameh

5. Har Har Har Har Gobinday
Har Har Har Har Mukanday
Har Har Har Har Udhaaray
Har Har Har Har Apaaray
Har Har Har Har Hareeung
Har Har Har Har Kareeung
Har Har Har Har Nirnaamay
Har Har Har Har Akaamay

6. Rakhay rakhanahaar aap ubaariun
Gur kee pairee paa-eh kaaj savaariun
Hoaa aap dayaal manho na visaariun
Saadh janaa kai sung bhavjal taariun
Saakat nindak dusht khin maa-eh bidaariun
Tis saahib kee tayk Naanak manai maa-eh
Jis simrat sukh ho-eh saglay dookh jaa-eh

Thou who savest, save us all and take us across,
Uplifting and giving the excellence.
You gave us the touch of the lotus feet of the Guru, and all our jobs are done.
You have become merciful, kind, and compassionate; and so our mind does not forget Thee.
In the company of the holy beings you take us from misfortune and calamities, scandals, and disrepute. Godless, slanderous enemies—you finish them in timelessness. That great Lord is my anchor.
Nanak, keep firm in your mind, by meditating and repeating His Name all happiness comes and all sorrows and pain go away.

Later, he gave some optional mudras to use with this sadhana in order to increase prosperity. In the second chant, you may sit with the hands crossed over each other at the center of the chest. In the third chant—the Mul Mantra—alternate the arms with each repetition in the following manner: Extend the arms forward, parallel to the ground, both palms up with right hand resting in the left. For the next repetition hold the arms straight up, palms together in Prayer Pose above the head, arms hugging the ears. For the next repetition extend them straight ahead as before but with the left hand resting in the right. Continue in this pattern throughout the chant. During the fourth chant, sit with the palms together in Prayer Pose at the center of the chest; as you begin each phrase of the mantra, extend the arms smoothly up and forward to a 60° angle. Bring them back quickly to the Heart Center to begin the next phrase. During the fifth mantra, bring the hands in front of the Navel Point, palms facing each other. In a steady pulse, as you chant *Har*, move your hands toward each other and away four times and then hold them still during the last word of each line of the chant, for example, *Gobinday*. During the last mantra, place your left hand on the Heart Center and bring your right hand, in Gyan Mudra, up beside the shoulder, with the elbow relaxed down.

The Aquarian Sadhana

From the very beginning, Yogi Bhajan talked about the grand transition and maturation of human beings that would mark the Aquarian Age. Everything he taught us was to prepare us for this transition in the year 2012. After that we will begin to see all that he envisioned. We will need intuition, stamina, both physical and mental, self-awareness, and a new depth of spiritual experience that can hold our identity in the face of global changes, relentless competition, information overload, and ecological and environmental challenges.

He gave us the Aquarian Sadhana in 1992 to take us through this transition period and to prepare our psyches to excel in the new environments in the decades after 2012. He envisioned an end to the world as we think of it now—not an end to the world. What sadhana can give us the awareness, the fearlessness, the compassion, kindness, and the spirit to serve, teach and prosper no matter what changes happen within in us and around us? The Aquarian Sadhana. This meditation series is the contemplative technology to master your mind and prepare your consciousness for the new Age. He asked us to practice it worldwide until 2012 and beyond; it could be practiced throughout the Aquarian Age. It attunes your *gunas*, your chakras and your mind to the change of the Age. After 2012, we can practice it or any of the other sadhanas he shared. And just as he changed or adjusted the practice of sadhana over the years to match the needs of the time, now KRI and the continuing legacy of teachers in the tradition of Kundalini Yoga as taught by Yogi Bhajan® will share the teachings and guide the use and application of them to match up to the new opportunities and needs.

The total time for this sequence of mantras is 62 minutes. They can be done with any meditative musical melody that preserves the *Naad* and rhythm of the mantras. Only one mantra requires a specific posture and mudra.

I. Morning Call: (7 minutes)
Ek Ong Kaar, Sat Naam Siree, Wha-hay Guroo

The cornerstone of this morning sadhana is the Adi Shakti Mantra, also called Long Ek Ong Kars or Morning Call. This mantra awakens the kundalini, initiating the relationship between our soul and the Universal Soul.

Long Ek Ong Kars are chanted without musical accompaniment, whereas the six mantras that follow may be chanted using various melodies with or without instrumental accompaniment. (Musicians take note: instruments are for background to accompany and support the voice. Also, be sure to preserve the original rhythm of the mantra by keeping the length of the syllables intact.)

2. Waah Yantee (7 Minutes)
Waah Yantee, Kar Yantee, Jagat Utpatee,
Aadak It Whaa-haa, Brahmaaday Trayshaa Guroo
It Wha-hay Guroo

3. The Mul Mantra: (7 minutes)
Ek Ong Kaar, Sat Naam, Kartaa Purakh,
Nirbho Nirvair, Akaal Moort, Ajoonee Saibhang,
Gurprasaad. Jap.
Aad Such Jugad Such Haibhee Such
Naanak Hosee Bhee Such

The Mul Mantra gives an experience of the depth and consciousness of your soul. In chanting the Mul Mantra leave a slight space (not a breath) between ajoonee and saibhang. Do not run the words together. Emphasize the "ch" sound at the end of the word "such."

4. Sat Siri, Siri Akal (7 minutes)

Yogi Bhajan has called this the Mantra for the Aquarian Age, with it we declare that we are timeless, deathless beings:

Sat Siree	*Great Truth*
Siree Akaal	*Great beyond Death*
Siree Akaal	*Great beyond Death*
Maahaa Akaal	*Great beyond Death*
Maahaa Akaal	*Great beyond Death*
Sat Naam	*Truth identified (Named)*
Akaal Moorat	*Truth is His Name*
Wha-hay Guroo	*Great Beyond Words is his Wisdom*

5. Rakhe Rakhanhar (7 minutes)

Rakhay rakhanahaar aap ubaariun
Gur kee pairee paa-eh kaaj savaariun
Hoaa aap dayaal manho na visaariun
Saadh janaa kai sung bhavjal taariun
Saakat nindak dusht khin maa-eh bidaariun
Tis saahib kee tayk Naanak manai maa-eh
Jis simrat sukh ho-eh saglay dookh jaa-eh

6.Wha-hay Guroo Wha-hay Guroo Wha-hay Guroo Wha-hay Jeeo (22 minutes)

Great beyond description is His Infinite Wisdom.

Sit in Virasan, on the left heel, with the right foot flat on the floor and the knee drawn in toward the chest. The hands are in Prayer Pose at the Heart Center and the eyes are at the tip of the nose.

7. Guru Ram Das Chant (5 minutes)
Guroo Guroo Wha-hay Guroo
Guroo Raam Das Guroo

A Spectrum of Other Sadhanas

During these same years where general sadhana guidelines were given by Yogi Bhajan, he also gave special sadhanas, some independent from these core practices, some to combine with them for a particular purpose and some to create a targeted effect for a short time.

Raaga Meditation Sadhana

In 1998 Sangeet Kaur & Harjinder Singh put together an Aquarian Sadhana CD for the meditations using rhythms and scales in the classical raag of Indian music. Yogi Bhajan used the release of this new album as an opportunity to give us a raaga sadhana to balance the mind, aura and electromagnetic field. He gave it as 40-day practice and challenged his students to test it by experience. He commented: "I want you to do it for 40 days, in the morning, and go through it. When you polarize your energy and electromagnetic seal of your body, you will understand your head needs something across your heart. It is not difficult to do. But at least you will not be spaced out and talking to angels—you will become an angel."

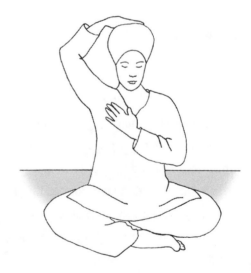

Mudra: Sit in Easy Pose with a straight spine. Left hand: Bring the left palm flat against the chest with the wrist at the Heart Center, the rest of the hand is angled at 60° with the fingers pointing toward the right shoulder. Right hand: Bring the right hand, palm flat and face down over the crown of the head—the 10th gate. The elbow will be bent slightly. Hold the position steady. Eyes: Stare at the tip of the nose through closed eyes.

Music: Raaga Sadhana by Sangeet Kaur & Harjinder Singh. Play it from the beginning and chant along with it. To End: Inhale deep, press the hand against the heart, hold the breath and distribute the energy in your being. Hold 15-20 seconds. Exhale. Inhale deeply, press the hand against the heart, distribute the energy; hold the breath 10-15 seconds. Exhale. Inhale a third time and bring the right palm on top of the left palm at your Heart Center. Press very firmly with all your will, hold the breath tight, and let the energy spread. Hold for 20-25 seconds. Cannon Fire the breath out through your mouth. Relax.

Evening Sadhanas

During the 1980s, Yogi Bhajan gave us several evening sadhanas to increase the power of protection and guidance through hard or chaotic times of change. These were done in addition to the morning sadhanas. In 1983 he gave us the following evening sadhana:

1. *Har Har Har Har Har Har Haree for 11 minutes.*

Chant powerfully in a monotone from the Navel Point, keeping the mouth slightly open, but not moving the lips. Use the tongue. Keep the eyes at the tip of the nose. Sit in Virasan on the right heel, hands grasping opposite biceps at shoulder level. Left foot on the ground pulled close to the body with the left knee up near the chest.

2. *Chant this mantra for one hour: Aap Sahaee Hoaa Sachay Daa Sachay Dhoaa Har Har Har*

In 1984 he extended the evening sadhana into three parts:

1. *Har Har Har Har Har Har Haree* for 22 minutes. Sit on the right heel, hands holding the opposite biceps with the eyes at the tip of the nose. Left foot flat on the ground near the body with the left knee raised close to the chest.

2. *Aap Sahaee Hoaa Sachay Daa Sachay Dhoaa Har Har Har for 22 minutes*

Sit in a meditative pose. No focus was specified.

3. *Chant for 22 minutes:*
Chattr Chakkr Vartee
Chattre Chakkr Bhugatay
Suyambhav Subhang Sarb Daa Sarb Jugtay,
Dukaalang Pranaasee Dayaalang Sarroopay
Sadaa Ung Sungay Abhangang Bibhootay

Thou art pervading in all the four directions,
The Enjoyer in all the four directions.
Thou art self-illumined and united with all.
Destroyer of bad times, embodiment of mercy,
Thou art ever within us.
Thou art the everlasting giver of indestructible power.

These are the last few lines of *Jaap Sahib*, written by Guru Gobind Singh, one of the world's greatest yogis and teachers. To chant this sit in Virasan: sit on the left heel, hands in Prayer Pose. Right foot on the ground close to body and the right knee bent close to the chest.

This is a powerful practice. It can help conquer almost any fear and open your vision for a way forward.

Kirtan Kriya Sadhana

In the 1970s when he first taught Kirtan Kriya, one of the core practices of Kundalini Yoga, he gave a way to practice it as a sadhana. Prepare for a 40-day sadhana of chanting Kirtan Kriya for 2½ hours in half hour cycles (refer to the description of Kirtan Kriya on page 148). During this 40-day period, wear all white. If possible, create a sacred meditation space with a small altar that is white in all aspects. Make your diet very light and eat only vegetables and grains, with some milk or yogurt as necessary. Never eat until full. Drink plenty of fluids. Be aware of your speech and only use words that are conscious, kind and harmonious.

This is an example of a sadhana practice that is based on the effect of one meditation kriya. The 40 days maximizes the kriya's effect to clear the subconscious and create a habit of awareness. This will give you a different experience than the balanced sadhanas with the medley of mantras that we do in a group sadhana. It is an excellent discipline that allows one to gradually master certain core kriyas through this type of focused effort. Over time it gives you a wide spectrum of capacities and experiences.

In a similar manner we did 40 days of the Adi Shakti mantra or 40 days of the Guru Gaitri mantra—each for 2½ hours. We usually did a bit of yoga before the extended meditation and we always followed with shivasana, a lay-out.

Shabd Guru: Sadhana through the Divine Sound Current

Yogi Bhajan also shared with us the unique sadhana that is the legacy of the yogis and gurus of the Sikh tradition. The sadhana is based in the repetition of the mantras and *shabds* of the Siri Guru Granth Sahib. This unique composition of sacred writings and mantra was designed to convey the living consciousness and presence of the great masters and of the divine within each of us. When a student reads continuously from the passages of the Siri Guru Granth Sahib, the sound current of the passages confronts the mind with the consciousness of your spirit and you soul. The Siri Guru Granth Sahib acts as a teacher; it is a living interaction—a relationship with your spirit—that clarifies the mind and opens the heart. Yogi Bhajan shared many different ways in which to read and relate to the sound current: read a single passage, read the continuous sound current for an hour or more, or participate with others to create a continuous reading of the entire scripture over a period of three days to a week, known as an Akhand Path. Engaging in the sound current, the Siri Guru Granth Sahib, is a very unique and enjoyable technique once you realize that it is not about learning any particular content or idea. This sadhana is about raising your awareness of the interaction between your mind and your soul. The energy put into the words of this sacred composition by the Saints, Gurus and Yogis who composed it creates a mirror through which one can see one's own life and existence. With great love and clarity it touches your heart and gives you the opportunity to put aside ego and to let in the vastness and the wonder of this creation and its Creator. Sikhs, Hindus, Muslims and others have contributed to this unique scripture; its deepest value comes from the accuracy and authenticity with which it expresses the experience of that state of consciousness that the writer was in when it was written—being one with God.

As you recite it, a spark of that energy and awareness comes into you as the reader. The particular rhythms and combinations of sounds guide not only your thoughts but also your neurology; you begin to function on a higher level. This universal technology of the sound current is open to all and has become a steadfast part of the legacy of consciousness that is our practice of Kundalini Yoga. Guru Ram Das, a great Yogi as well as a Guru, was acknowledged to hold the throne of healing for the Raj Yoga of awareness; this Raj Yoga is at the core of our identity as Kundalini Yogis and Teachers, serving all in the Aquarian Age.

Steps Toward an Ideal Sadhana

Even the thought of doing sadhana is the beginning of sadhana. Our actions and commitments start with a thought, with a feeling in our heart, some small seed of desire. Here are some models of how to do an ideal sadhana in the 2½ hours before the rise of the Sun and some steps toward that for beginners. Whether your sadhana consists of 10 minutes of prayer, an hour of exercise, 31 minutes of a powerful kriya, an hour of reading the divine sound current or the full 2½ hours of traditional sadhana, you will experience immediate benefits and project an increased radiance throughout your day. The most important thing is to begin.

Sadhana is a discipline by which we show up before our Self to do the maintenance that our physical body needs for good health and vitality and to confront, clear and qualify our mind, clearing out the garbage so that we can rest the mind in the sound current and project from neutrality in any given situation throughout our day. These models give you a basic structure around which you can tailor your own practice. The ideal remains a full 2½-hour sadhana before the rise of the sun. We've provided a sample timeline in the Aquarian Sadhana; these times remain fairly consistent throughout all the models unless otherwise indicated.

The Aquarian Sadhana

This is the sadhana that Yogi Bhajan gave us to practice through the year 2012. Already discussed above, the following is a sample timeline for this practice. Meant to be a model for morning sadhana only, we've given a range of start times for each section; they are approximate and may be adjusted according to the needs of the group. The length of time for each mantra meditation is fixed and should not be altered. When you lead a group sadhana be sure to have clear beginning and ending times to allow everyone to coordinate and to feel welcomed into the experience.

A note to Sadhana Leaders: The first guideline for sadhana leaders is show up! If you are leading, be there first and on time. Whenever possible have a designated back-up leader to cover the sadhana if there is some reason you must be absent. Always respect the space of sadhana as a sacred duty not a personal performance.

Sample Schedule

3:00-3:15am Begin wake-up and preparation for sadhana

3:45-4:00am Optional Recitation of *Japji Sahib*

If you are unfamiliar with *Japji* or concerned about pronunciation, use a tape or CD. When possible, read *Japji* in the call and answer form—tantric style—male-female reading alternate lines. A copy of *Japji*, in English, gurmukhi or as an mp3 can be downloaded from http://sikhnet.com

4:00-4:20am Tune In. Begin with the Adi Mantra: Ong Namo Guru Dev Namo.

4:05-4:45am Kundalini Yoga Kriya for 25-45 minutes.

As the leader, be sensitive to the environment and establish one conducive to sadhana. Adjust lights, noises, temperature and other factors. There will always be individual differences; find the happy medium that will serve the group as a whole. The yoga kriya should include exercises that enhance flexibility, stretching and pranayam. Many kriyas are provided for you here; there are also numerous manuals with clearly documented exercises available from KRI. Music can be played during the kriyas, but most find that these early morning hours of meditation and exercise are best served by silence, unless the kriya calls for a particular selection of music to support the movement of the energy.

4:45am Deep Relaxation

Dim the lights as needed. Participants can lie down in corpse pose or sit meditatively. Keep the relaxation relatively short—as brief as 3 minutes, average about 5 minutes or possibly a little more, but always under 10 minutes—according to the kriyas chosen. You want people to rest in *yoga nidra* not lapse into a long dreaming sleep. This can be in silence or with meditative mantra music played softly. Come out of the relaxation by rotating the wrists and ankles; then rapidly rub the palms of the hands and the soles of the feet together. Cat stretch four or five times, left and right. Pull the knees to the chest and rock back and forth to massage the length of the spine.

5:00am The Aquarian Sadhana Mantra Meditations. 62 minutes.

Lights can be turned very low or completely off. Keep sadhana music, live or recorded, loud enough to be heard clearly throughout the entire sadhana room, so that it envelops the participants, and is easy to sing along with. The music supports the recitation. Let the music surround and expand you. You could also do some or all of the mantras *a capella* or without accompaniment. The focus is to engage the mind in the sound current and dwell in the energy of the mantra as you process the flow of thoughts and feelings.

6:00am Concluding Contemplative Moments.

Spend a few moments of deep listening and silence followed by an inspirational reading, a prayer or a selection from *Japji* or the Siri Guru Granth Sahib. Then sing May The Long Time Sun Shine Upon You to project light, healing and prayers to all.

6:15-6:30am Close of Sadhana.

For those who know the art and science of taking a *hukam* from the Guru, this is an appropriate time.

A Basic Model of Sadhana

• Wake-up and preparation for sadhana

• Optional Recitation of Japji Sahib

• Tune In with the Adi Mantra:
  Ong Namo Guru Dev Namo.

• Pranayam for 10 minutes

• Kundalini Yoga Kriya for 30-45 minutes.

• Deep Relaxation for 5-7 minutes; coming out in the usual manner. (See Aquarian Sadhana)

• Begin Kundalini Yoga Chants for 62 minutes or less. Choose from the following options:

The Adi Shakti Mantra or Morning Call:
Ek Ong Kar, Sat Nam Siri, Wahe Guru.

If this is the only mantra you use in the morning then chant for a minimum of 37½ minutes. (There is an mp3 available from kriteachings.org to aid you in this practice.)

• • •

Chant the Laya Yoga form of the Adi Shakti Mantra:
Ek Ong Kar-uh Sat Naam-uh Siree Wha-uh Hay Guroo for 31 minutes, followed by 10–15 minutes of long **Sat Nam**

• • •

The Panj Shabad: **Sa Ta Na Ma** for 31 minutes (please see Kirtan Kriya on p. 148) followed by 31 minutes of the Adi Shakti Mantra (Morning Call).

• • •

Chant the Adi Shakti Mantra (Morning Call) for 31 minutes followed by 31 minutes of the Guru Gaitri Mantra: **Gobinday, Mukanday, Udaaray, Apaaray, Hareeung, Kareeung, Nirnaamay, Akaamay**

62

- Sit in Silence for 5-10 minutes. Then lie down to relax again for 3-10 minutes. Come out of relaxation in the usual manner.

- Meditate on the healing energy of Guru Ram Das by chanting Guru Guru Wahe Guru Guru Ram Das Guru for several minutes.

- Concluding Contemplative Moments: Spend a few moments of deep listening and silence followed by an inspirational reading, prayer or a selection from *Japji* or the Siri Guru Granth Sahib Then sing May The Long Time Sun Shine Upon You to project light, healing and prayers to all.

Pranayam and Meditation Sadhana

In this practice, many of the elements are the same; however, the focus is on the breath and meditation rather than a long exercise set:

- Wake-up, Preparation and Tune-in

- Pranayam: choose a powerful pranayam practice for 15-20 minutes.

- Warm-up and a short, vigorous kriya for 10-15 minutes

- Meditation: choose a meditation and practice for up to 15 minutes

- Relaxation for 3-10 minutes

- Chant up to 62 minutes: You can choose to use the Aquarian Sadhana chants or from the other Kundalini Chants offered in the Basic Model of Sadhana.

- Silence: 10-15 minutes

- Close with Long Time Sun along with other contemplative readings or prayers.

Mastering the Kriya Sadhana

This sadhana focuses on mastering a particular kriya as well as exploring a wide range of kriyas. It's a great model for those who want to increase their fitness level on the physical plane as well as increase their nerve strength and support their detoxification process.

On your own, or as a community, choose a kriya that you'd like to master. Typically it will be a kriya that calls for 7-11 minutes for each exercise and recommends increasing a few minutes each day until the kriya can be practiced with the full times. A good example is Nabhi Kriya. Here's what this sadhana would look like:

- Wake-up, Preparation, and Tune-in

- Warm-ups and Pranayam for 15-30 minutes

- Kriya for Mastery: This is the exercise set that you have chosen to master. Practice it each day for 11, 40, 90, or 120 days—or until mastery is achieved. Remember to start slowly and gradually increase the times each day until you can complete each exercise in the kriya for the full times indicated.

- Silent Meditation for 3-10 minutes

- Kriya Exploration: Choose a different kriya every day; make sure that it can be practiced in under 15 minutes. This is a great opportunity to explore many of the shorter kriyas that Yogi Bhajan outlined for us, for example, Varuyas Kriya or Disease Resistance and Heart Helper.

- Silent Meditation for 3-10 minutes

- End this kriya portion of the sadhana with moderate exercises in which all the limbs have a chance to move; you could even dance to soft meditative music.

- Chant for up to 62 minutes choosing from the models outlined

- Silence: 10-15 minutes

- Close with Long Time Sun along with other contemplative readings or prayers.

The Student-Teacher Sadhana

Yogi Bhajan said that this should be done once or twice a year by every student-teacher. This model focuses on the chanting of the *Nam* using the Adi Shakti Mantra, other core mantra from the Kundalini Yoga tradition, or the Siri Guru Granth Sahib.

The Adi Shakti Mantra, or Morning Call—should be the first choice because it is the fundamental Kundalini mantra. Forty days of this practice provides a transformation and cleansing beyond price. If you decide to do a second 2 ½ hour sadhana using the *Nam*, explore another core mantra or the depth and beauty of reading from the Siri Guru Granth Sahib. Here's what this practice would look like:

- Wake-up, Preparation, and Tune-in

- Short kriya to open the hips and prepare you to sit.

- Chant for 2 ½ hours with steady, sonorous, clear tones.

- Meditate silently on the sound for 5 minutes.

- Relax for 15 minutes.

- Close with a few minutes of Guru Guru Wahe Guru, Guru Ram Das Guru, other contemplative readings or prayers, and finally, May the Long Time Sun Shine song.

VARIATION: Sometimes it is impossible to do the 2 ½

hours of chanting all in the morning. Yogi Bhajan said we can split the chanting into two parts if necessary. In this case, it is best to chant for 1 ½ hours both morning and evening.

Anahat Sadhana: Into the Subtle Current of Naad

There are times when you need to practice deep silent meditation on the *Nam*. Yogi Bhajan said that the prime hour for this type of meditation is between 2:30 and 3:30 a.m., the calmest time of the day. The inner sound current is loudest at this time. A simple alteration of the sadhana schedule can accommodate your practice at that time.

- Wake-up, Preparation, and Tune-in

- Beginning at 2:30 am, meditate for 45 minutes to an hour. Sit in deep stillness and listen with the inner ear as well as the outer. Listen to the inner sound current with a meditative breath, as slow as one breath per minute. Let the heard and unheard pulse of the *Naad* vibrate in every cell of the body and dwell in absolute, sustained stillness and awareness.

- Kriya for 31 minutes to an hour.

- Chant for up to 62 minutes

- Deep Relaxation for 5-20 minutes

- Close with a prayer, reading, or hukam and Long Time Sun to bless yourself and bless the world.

A Beginner's Sadhana

This is an example of how you might start building a morning practice if you have had little experience and you want to increase your time commitment slowly.

This takes about one hour a day and will give you energy and balance. Change the kriyas every few weeks. Increase the time gradually, moving toward the complete Aquarian Sadhana.

• Wake-up, Preparation, and Tune-in

• Kriya for 15-31 minutes: Choose three short exercise sets 15–31 minutes each. Select a combination that works on different areas and systems of your body. Alternate these sets in a three-day pattern, doing one kriya per day so that on the fourth day you begin again with the first kriya. In this way, no muscles become too sore and each part of your system gets a thorough workout over the course of the week.

• Relaxation for 5-10 minutes.

• Chant the Adi Shakti Mantra (Morning Call) for 31 minutes or select a meditation that fits your needs.

• Close with a prayer and Long Time Sun to bless yourself and bless the world.

Legacy—A Sadhana from the Early Days of 3HO

We include this in our many models of sadhana in order to honor the way we began and continue the legacy of the first foundations of sadhana that Yogi Bhajan taught. It begins by tuning into the Golden Chain as we chant the Adi Mantra. We awaken, become humble, present and alert. Next is the Adi Shakti mantra—the fundamental mantra to awaken kundalini. This is followed by Sat Kriya to give strength, endurance and balance the lower three chakras. After the naval point is strengthened, the Guru Gaitri mantra (also known as the Sarab Shakti mantra) consolidates our energy and grants protection throughout the aura. The chanting finishes with the Kundalini Bhakti mantra establishing a relationship to our feminine and

the flow of kundalini energy throughout our life. The energy that is released and gathers within us from the chanting is distributed throughout the body and the nervous system with a vigorous exercise set. It concludes with a moment of intentional consciousness in which we put ourself before our higher self and offer a prayer, a spiritual reading or a selection from *Peace Lagoon*, an early translation of *Japji Sahib*. And as always, end with the 3HO blessing to all "May the long time sun shine upon you... ". We would then take time to do kirtan or sing uplifting songs as a group with all those who joined us to do morning sadhana. Here's the summary of this early practice:

• Wake-up, Preparation, Tune-In

• Chant the Adi Shakti mantra or Morning Call for 15 minutes: *Ek Ong Kaar, Sat Naam Siree, Wha-hay Guroo*

• Chant the Guru Gaitri Mantra mantra for 15 minutes: *Gobinday, Mukanday, Udaaray, Apaaray, Hareeung, Kareeung, Nirnaamay, Akaamay.*

• Chant the Kundalini Bhakti mantra for 15 minutes:
Aadee Shaktee, Aadee Shaktee, Aadee Shaktee,
Namo Namo
Sarab Shaktee, Sarab Shaktee, Sarab Shaktee,
Namo Namo
Pritham Bhaagavatee, Pritham Bhaagavatee,
Pritham Bhaagavatee,
Namo Namo
Kundalini Mata Shaktee, Mata Shaktee,
Namo Namo

I bow to the Primal Power.
I bow to the All Encompassing Power and Energy.
I bow to that through which God Creates.
I bow to the creative power of the kundalini,
the Divine Mother Power.

• Kriya: Vigorous Kundalini Yoga set for 30 minutes.

- Contemplative Closing: Take time to contemplate a selection from sacred writings such as *Peace Lagoon*, shabds from the Guru, the Siri Guru Granth Sahib, or others and close by blessing yourself and others with May the Long Time Sun.

- Enjoy singing or kirtan with all those who shared your sadhana or by yourself.

Special Intensives or Retreats

In addition to these models for morning sadhana, special retreats or focused intensives are forms of sadhana that enrich our lives, build communities and deepen our spiritual experience. Yogi Bhajan guided 3HO to create community gatherings at which we do intensive sadhanas, share experiences and resources, and simply celebrate life. The gathering times are usually the summer and winter solstice. These occur in North America, Latin America and various places in Europe.

White Tantra as Sadhana

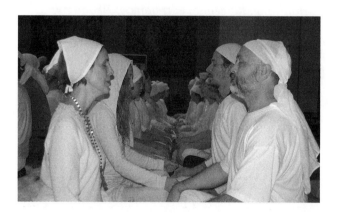

A very special and a powerful part of the legacy of the teachings of Yogi Bhajan is White Tantric Yoga. This intensive all-day experience is presented in one- or three-day courses. It is the fastest way to clear the subconscious and get rid of any fears. It is a profound way to induce healing in the body, mind and spirit. Yogi Bhajan would teach these intensive courses as a central experience during the solstice gatherings, as well as independently, as courses that gave people the opportunity to clear their minds and their karmas throughout the year. We encourage all students to participate in a sadhana that includes a White Tantric Yoga experience regularly. Participation in at least one White Tantric Meditation is required in order to become a Kundalini Yoga Teacher. There is a well-established worldwide circuit of White Tantra Yoga courses that you can find and participate in. See www.whitetantricyoga.com.

Becoming a Model of Sadhana

At first we do sadhana. Eventually, we become sadhana. At that point, the sadhana that we do each morning infuses every breath and every step of our day, seamlessly, with lightness, awareness and excellence. Sadhana becomes a consciousness and an identity, not just an activity.

The first step is always to begin where you are. Assess yourself, your level of commitment, your intention and your knowledge. If you are near a yoga center or ashram, join them for group sadhana. If you are by yourself, then begin a personal practice. You can form a small group, a few people, who join together to amplify each other's efforts in the early morning or during an evening sadhana. It is often said that on the spiritual path, if you take one step toward your higher consciousness or toward the guru then the guru takes a thousand steps toward you. Take heart, take the first step! Keep up!

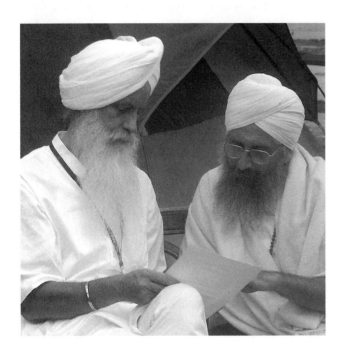

Question: Should I change the exercises and kriyas every day?

Answer: One part of the sadhana should stay constant long enough for you to master, or at least experience the changes evoked by a single technique. Each kriya and mantra has its individuality. Their effects are not all the same although they all levitate you toward a cosmic consciousness.

You may want to practice a spectrum of the many things Yogi Bhajan has shared with us. But at some point, stop window shopping and commit considerable attention and effort to one thing. Learn to value one kriya as priceless and all others will be understood in a clearer light. There is a natural 40-day rhythm to

habits in the body and mind. It takes about 40 days of consistent practice to break a habit. To establish a new habit in action and in the subconscious takes about 90 days. It is good to take these biorhythms into account when designing the sadhana for long-term results.

At least twice a year each teacher should accomplish a 40-day, 2½-hour sadhana of either chanting the 2½ breath, Long Ek Ong Kar mantra (Morning Call), or reading from the Siri Guru Granth Sahib.

Question: Is leading sadhana the same as teaching a class?

Answer: No. There are differences. No matter where you teach a class of exercises, it will be 60 minutes or less, including relaxation. But in sadhana, there is regular attendance which allows everyone to focus on a particular kriya and gradually increase the length of practice. In a class, you might chant long Sat Nam for 7–10 minutes; in sadhana you could build it up to 31 or 45 minutes. Another difference is the amount of talking that should be done. In an outside class, there is more need for inspiring, coaxing and explaining. Sadhana occurs in the quiet, ambrosial hours. We should speak only of the Infinite, and mostly we should listen to the Infinite.

Question: If I have to leave sadhana, what is the best way?

Answer: The same way you entered. Be aware of the presence of the teacher by bowing in your consciousness.

Be quiet so nothing is disturbed. Choose a time to leave that is between kriyas and meditations. A sharp noise during a deep meditation is a shock to the total system. Do not come and go as you please, but as would please the highest teacher.

Question: Should I wake someone up who falls asleep in sadhana?

Answer: No. God should wake him. The experience of sadhana is between the individual and God. Do not interfere. You can inspire beforehand. If sleeping is a chronic habit, discuss it with the person at a convenient time, but do not abruptly wake someone. He may be at a different level of experience than you think. It is our intention, of course, to stay totally alert and awake.

Question: When I am sick, should I attend sadhana?

Answer: If you are going to be in bed all day with an extreme sickness, then no. If it is not extreme, then attend sadhana and do what you can. If you cannot exercise, then at least attempt to meditate. Afterwards, lie down and rest in sadhana while mentally listening to the *shabd*. This way you will get well faster and maintain the rhythm of a regular sadhana. It also eliminates the tendency to have minor morning illnesses to escape the self-discipline of a constant sadhana. In other words, participation in a group effort and regularity of discipline are paramount, but do not be a fanatic to the point of aggravating a serious illness.

Question: Can I do an individual sadhana?

Answer: It is fine anytime in the day that does not interfere with your commitments. That period of time before group sadhana begins is excellent. If you have a special health sadhana that you must do as an as-

signed yogic therapy by your teacher then you can do that. However, the general rule is that individual sadhana is not a substitute for group sadhana. A primary goal of sadhana is to develop the group consciousness into a universal consciousness. It requires a conscious intention backed-up by regular practice to create a habit to give morning sadhana and group sadhana a priority.

Question: I am a beginner and can only spend one hour on sadhana. Will one hour have any affect?

Answer: Always do some sadhana no matter how short, for every effort of the individual mind to meet the Universal Self is reciprocated a thousand-fold. The ideal is a perfect 2½-hour sadhana. But if we are to run, we must first learn to walk. An hour is an excellent beginner's sadhana. As you grow in your sadhana, you will find time to extend it if you really want to do so. It is good for some people to start more slowly. If you try to climb Mt. Everest without climbing even a foothill beforehand, failure could discourage you from all other attempts. Build slowly and constantly at a pace you can maintain, but definitely do something!

Question: As the leader of sadhana, should I participate in all the exercises?

Answer: As a leader, your responsibility is to set a good example and to give clear instructions for each step of the sadhana. You should do as many exercises as you can without becoming unaware of the group. You must check to make sure that everyone is doing the exercise properly before beginning yourself. Sometimes it will be better not to participate at all. Always join in during chanting. When teaching a class outside of sadhana, you should participate as little as possible in the physical exercise. Concentrate only on inspiring and serving the class.

Question: When chanting in the morning, the pitch

often gets low. What, if anything, should be done to change the pitch?

Answer: Chant at a constant, mid-range pitch as much as possible. If your breath rhythm is not correct, or your spine is not kept straight, or you do not take complete breaths in the Adi Shakti Mantra, the mantra will lose energy and drop in pitch. If you project the sound of the mantra from the back of the mouth in a full and round way, the power of the chant will increase as you continue and the pitch will stay constant.

If you are constant and listen to the sound of your chant, you will hear different pitches. These are actually overtones of the basic sound you are creating. The overtones will be high-pitched, subtle and seem to float around the room. You cannot identify that tone with one person since it is formed by the combination of group sounds. The overtone is a good sign that the sadhana group is tuned in to each other and beyond each other. As you listen to the first overtone and become very calm, you may begin to hear even higher and more subtle overtones. This awareness aids meditation on the etheric echo of your chanting as you sit silently after chanting aloud.

If your group is united in consciousness, no one will shift the pitch. If the pitch does shift, it will seem to do so by itself. It will shift smoothly and infrequently.

Question: Is it all right to harmonize with the main tone?

Answer: Chanting is not singing. It is vibrating all the cells of the body, all the thoughts of the mind and the core crystal of the soul to the same shabd. Chanting in meditation is beyond personality. Chanting like a choir with many harmonies turns the group consciousness, which is striving for universality, into individual consciousness responding to social consciousness. Leave vocal harmonizing for kirtan and other musical gatherings. Learn to harmonize the body, mind, and soul while chanting.

Question: Are there different sadhanas for different days of the week?

Answer: Each day of the week has its own energy. In astrology this is symbolized by associating each day with a planet. (See the chart on page 70 for all the qualities.) The daily sadhana exercise series could be chosen to relate to these energies. An emotional, calming pranayam for Monday; a nabhi (Navel Point) kriya for Tuesday; a brain cleansing set for Wednesday; a deep meditation Thursday; a sex transmutation series Friday; a strenuous physical cleansing kriya Saturday; and a blissful projective Laya Yoga meditation Sunday. This is a good idea, but if you are varying the sadhana exercise daily, you will also find that each day of the week differs from week to week. Ultimately you must use your own sensitivity to choose what kind of energy to deal with in the exercises. The chart may be used as a guide.

Question: Should I bring my children to sadhana?

Answer: Your children are the future. The future will only be as secure as the foundation that is built into the young generation. It is very inspirational to see the radiance from young children who attend the last portion of sadhana during chanting. Usually the young ones do not attend during exercises although very young ones may sleep through them and there is no restriction.

Whether or not your particular child should attend is an individual determination. If he has been raised in the yogic tradition where chanting and exercise are a natural part of his environment, then bring him. If he is very disruptive during sadhana, then his attendance should be discussed with the ashram family for a final decision.

Question: Is it important to wear a head covering?

Answer: During sadhana, be sure to cover your head with a non-static, natural cloth like cotton and keep the hair up. The hair regulates the inflow of sun energy into the body. To let the solar energy flow without obstruction, let the hair grow its full natural length and take good care of it. If this is done, the amount of energy that goes downward from the Seventh Chakra increases tremendously. The kundalini energy is activated by the radiant force of the solar plexus and moves upward in response to the solar energy coming down. This balances the body energy and maintains equilibrium.

If the hair is down, unkempt or uncovered so that it is electrically imbalanced, this natural process of raising the kundalini energy will be impeded. Every major spiritual tradition has covered the head, but reasons often get lost through the centuries.

Question: Do we need a special place for sadhana?

Answer: In the ashram or your residence, a special place or altar is ideal. The care you give the external environment is a sign and symbol to the mind of your intention. The outer reflects the inner. If the place of meditation is sloppy it usually means you do not value relating to that Infinite Self, or you value it but do not believe in it, or yourself. When traveling, do your best to bring the sense of sacredness with you to wherever you meditate. Some people use a portable meditation picture or incense to help induce this feeling.

DAY	PLANET	SYMBOL	QUALITY
Monday	Moon	☽	Emotional
Tuesday	Mars	♂	Energetic, Combative
Wednesday	Mercury	☿	Business, Communication
Thursday	Jupiter	♃	Expansion and Deep Thought
Friday	Venus	♀	Love, Sensuality
Saturday	Saturn	♄	Karma, Constriction, Discipline
Sunday	Sun	☉	Purity, Energy of Self

Tuning In

Before beginning a set or meditation always begin by Tuning In. This sequence will ready your mind to expand unto the Infinity.

The Adi Mantra: *Ong Namo Guru Dev Namo*

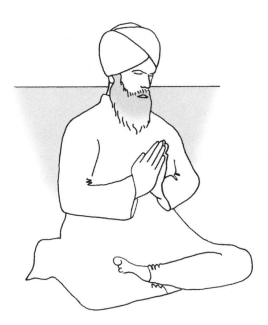

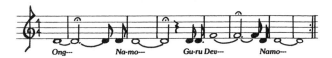

This mantra is chanted before every class or practice session involving Kundalini Yoga. If you read most old books about yoga, they say Kundalini Yoga is the most powerful of all yogas, but that it is dangerous. The fact is that if you practice it in the correct form, chant the universal *Nam*, and humble yourself before your higher Self or Teacher, it is perfectly safe. The Adi Mantra opens the protective channel of energy for Kundalini Yoga and brings you into the fold of the Golden Chain. It has been suggested that you should be able to visualize your Teacher seated over the crown of your head when reciting this mantra.

Ong is the infinite creative energy experienced in manifestation and activity. It is a variation of the cosmic syllable *Om* which is used to denote God in the absolute or unmanifested state. When God creates and functions as Creator, this is called *Ong*.

Namo has the same root as the word *Namaste* which means "reverent greetings." *Namaste* is a common form of respectful greeting in India accompanied by the mudra, Prayer Pose, either at the chest or forehead.

It implies bowing down. Together, *Ong Namo* means "I call on the infinite creative consciousness," opening yourself to the universal consciousness that guides all action.

Guru is the teacher or the embodiment of the wisdom that one is seeking. *Dev* means "divine" or "of God," in a non-earthly, transparent sense. *Namo*, in closing the mantra, reaffirms the humble reverence of the devotee. Taken together, *Guru Dev Namo* means "I call on the divine wisdom," in which you bow before your higher Self to guide you in using the knowledge and energy given by the cosmic self. To chant this mantra you should be sitting with a straight spine, with the palms of the hands joined so that the joints of the thumbs are at the sternum. The mantra is usually chanted at least three times. You inhale and chant *Ong Namo Guru Dev Namo* on one breath. Note that the sound *Dev* is chanted a minor third interval higher than the other sounds.

Ong Namo connects you to the Infinite that is beyond all and originates all forms. *Guru Dev Namo* connects you to the subtle intelligence that flows through all actions in life. The two parts of the mantra are a polarity that complete and balance each other.

There are some breathing exercises (pranayam), postures (asanas), hand positions (mudras), sound currents (mantra), and body locks (bandhs) that are used again and again in the practice of Kundalini Yoga. Become familiar with these basics by reading this section thoroughly and experiencing each pranayam, asana, mudra, and mantra. This will allow your practice of the kriyas to flow more smoothly and dynamically.

Pranayam

Kundalini Yoga employs a wide range of breathing techniques. They are more extensive and sophisticated than in any other form of yoga. The breath, its rhythm, and its depth are correlated to different states of health, consciousness, and emotion. Kundalini Yoga uses the breath scientifically to change the states of energy. By scientifically we mean that you can consistently produce a desired effect with regular practice. There are a few basic pranayams that should be mastered in order to freely practice the kriyas and meditations.

Long Deep Breath

The simplest of all the yogic breaths is just long deep breathing, but it is a habit that we, as a culture, do not have. Our normal tendency is to breathe irregularly and shallowly. This leads to a totally emotional approach to life, chronic tension, and weak nerves. The lungs are the largest internal organ of the human body. On average, lungs can enlarge to a volume of almost 6,000 cubic centimeters. Besides supplying oxygen to and removing carbon dioxide from the body, the respiratory system helps regulate body pH (acid/alkaline levels) and helps excrete water vapor,

hydrogen and small amounts of methane. Normally we may use only 600 or 700 cubic centimeters of that capacity. If you do not expand the lungs to their full capacity, the small air sacks in the lungs, called alveoli, cannot clean their mucous lining properly. Therefore you do not get enough oxygen and toxic irritants that lead to infections and disease build-up.

To take a full yogic breath you inhale by first relaxing the abdomen. Next expand the chest and finally the collarbones. As you exhale let the collarbones and chest deflate first, then pull the belly in completely. The diaphragm drops down to expand the lungs and contracts up to expel the air. As you inhale feel the back area of the lower ribs relax and expand. On the exhale be sure to keep the spine erect and steady; do not bend it or collapse the chest area. For some beginners, breathing is paradoxical; that is, instead of relaxing the navel on the inhalation, some breathe only into the upper chest as the navel pulls in toward the spine. Pay attention to the proper breath and paradoxical habits will give way to a natural energizing and cleansing breath.

For beginners: A good way to approach learning the natural breath is to lie down on your back with a phone book spread open across the navel. In this relaxed position, inhale and watch as the phone book rises; exhale and watch the book relax back down. It may take some time but patience pays and as this natural deep breath grows more familiar, you can begin practicing in Easy Sitting Pose with your hand on your navel. Again, observe the navel expand on the inhalation and draw back toward the spine on the exhalation.

By taking a deep yogic breath you can expand the lungs by about eight times. If you establish a habit of breathing long, deep, and slowly you will develop endurance and patience. If you can establish a breath rate of eight times per minute or less the pituitary starts secreting fully. If the breath is less than four times per minute the pineal gland starts functioning fully and deep meditation is automatic.

One Minute Breath

This is an extension of the Long Deep Breath practice and some kriyas and meditations will call for a One Minute Breath, so you will want to be familiar with it. In this breath, the inhalation is to the count of 20; then pause, suspending the breath for a count of 20; finally exhale to a count of 20. You can begin this practice by starting with smaller intervals: 8-8-8, 10-10-10 and so on, working your way up to the full One Minute Breath. It is said that in a conflict, the person who can breathe the slowest has the advantage. So this breath can serve you in more ways than one!

Breath of Fire

This breath is used consistently throughout Kundalini Yoga kriyas. It is very important that Breath of Fire be practiced and mastered by the student. In Breath of Fire, the focus of the energy is at the navel point. The breath is fairly rapid (2 to 3 breaths per second), continuous and powerful with no pause between the inhale and exhale. As you exhale, the air is pushed out by pulling the navel point and abdomen toward the spine. In this motion, the chest area remains fairly relaxed. The inhalation will occur naturally from the vacuum created by the exhale. This is a very balanced breath with no emphasis on either the exhale or the inhale, but rather equal power given to both. The inhale will feel easier than the exhale because the natural force of the diaphragm relaxing helps it.

Breath of Fire is a cleansing breath, renewing the blood and releasing old toxins from the lungs, mucous lining, blood vessels, and cells. It is a powerful way to adjust your autonomic nervous system and get rid of stress. Regular practice expands the lungs quickly. You can start with 3 minutes of Breath of Fire and build to

20 minutes. Begin by alternating 3 minutes of Breath of Fire with 2 minutes of rest for 5 complete sets of breath/relaxation.

Sitali Pranayam

This breath is often used to regulate fevers and blood pressure and to cure digestive ailments. To begin, curl the tongue and extend the tip just past the lips. Inhale deeply, drawing the breath in through the curled tongue. Exhale through the nose. (See Sitali Kriya, page 88).

Segmented Breathing

There is a wide range of segmented breaths used in Kundalini Yoga kriyas. A segmented breath is defined by the inhalation and exhalation being divided into sections, in specific ratios. Each ratio gives a different effect. Some typical ratios for inhale, hold, exhale, hold, are as follows: 1:4:2:0, 4:16:2:0, 4:0:1:0, and 1:8:1:8. As an example, examine the 4:0:1:0 ratio. This breath is used to heal oneself and to break depressions. You break the inhale into four equal sections. Each part is a quick, sniff-like inhale. Exhale in a single long stroke through the nose. It is important to focus on the flow of the breath and to keep the broken breath equally divided.

Whistle Breath

In this pranayam, you make a small hole with the lips, in a sense, puckering. Inhale and make a high-pitched whistle, then exhale through the nose. Another variation is to inhale through the nose and exhale with a whistle through the lips. Listen to the high-pitched sound as you breathe. This breathing changes the circulation and activates the higher glands such as the thyroid and parathyroid.

There are many other types of breathing but these are the basic elements of most breaths you will encounter.

Asanas

Variations on the Seated Posture

Asana means a posture consciously taken. Each asana has its own effect on awareness, reflexes and emotions. There are a great number of asanas used in the kriyas of Kundalini Yoga. Some are very easy to attain, others take gradual cultivation to master. Each exercise of a Kundalini Yoga kriya specifies what position to take. Sometimes the instruction for the seated posture in the exercise or meditation is not fixed. The requirement may be to sit in any meditative or cross-legged pose, or to sit in Easy Pose. In these cases the main requirement is for the spine to be straight and the posture to be balanced. Any of the sitting positions listed here would fit the requirements.

When you sit for meditation it is important that you feel balanced and stable. If you are leaning to one side or have great pain from the knees or ankles, you cannot meditate. If you do get into meditation in an off-balance posture you run the risk of misdirecting the energy and blood circulation that is stimulated by the kriya. Meditating in a chair, for example, is perfectly all right for those kriyas that allow it, but if you sit with the legs half dangling or with uneven pressure on the feet, then the blood distribution in the pelvis area will be imbalanced with respect to the two sides of the body. This in turn can offset the navel point which can lead to headaches, menstrual irregularity, digestive problems, and a host of minor pains whose causes are difficult to find.

Remember that the parts of the body are all interconnected and affect each other. Your posture should always feel well-balanced and comfortable to you. It should reflect harmony. In certain deep meditations your consciousness may alter to the degree that you temporarily lose your normal body awareness. In that case, the posture must be balanced in such a way that it is easy for the body to hold automatically without your conscious effort. If you are imbalanced then the muscles may jerk or spasm to adjust for stress. That little spasm can slightly rotate or displace a vertebra. When yoga was still new to this country, some entrepreneurs introduced meditation while doing the headstand. This was showy and tantalizingly different, but it led to many twisted necks and ruined meditations. With this in mind, choose any of the postures below and be conscious to set yourself well.

The surface you sit on must not be cold or too hard. That is why most yoga practitioners sit on a sheepskin or mat. A thick pad or large pillow doesn't work well because there is not enough support to stabilize the spine. A sheepskin is just the right thickness. It also provides an electromagnetic insulation from the ground. This prevents you from feeling tired or drained of energy as you meditate. The next best materials to sit on are wool, cotton, and silk. The worst surface to sit on is concrete or stone. Although you are designed with a natural pillow to sit on you still need to care for the spinal balance and electromagnetic integration of your nervous system.

Sukasana or Easy Pose

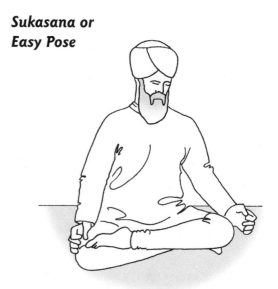

There are three variations of Sukasana which are commonly used in the exercises and meditation:

Variation One

Sit with the legs out straight. Pull the left foot into the groin. Place the right foot over the ankle of the left foot so that it rests near the thigh. Straighten the spine. This position can be done on the alternate side as well.

Variation Two

A delicate and effective variation is to assume Sukasana and then lift the heel of the foot near the groin. Bring it away from the body two or three inches. Arrange the foot on top so it rests directly on the calf with the ankle of the top foot about two inches up from the ankle of the bottom foot. In this pose make sure to press the lower spine forward. It will have a tendency to lose its natural, supporting curve.

Variation Three

If the first two postures are too strenuous for you then try this variation. Sit up with both legs straight. Put one foot under the opposite knee and then draw the extended foot under the other knee. Pull the spine up straight and press the lower spine slightly forward.

All of these poses require less flexibility and are easier on the knees than the Lotus Pose. The drawback is that you must be more conscious of keeping the lower spine slightly forward so the upper spine can stay straight.

Lotus Pose

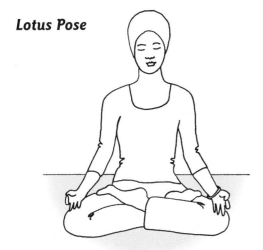

Sit with the legs extended forward. Spread the legs. Bend the left leg so the left heel comes to the groin.

Lift the left foot onto the upper right thigh. Bend the right leg so that the right foot goes over the left thigh as close to the abdomen as possible. Straighten the spine. Lift the chest and press the lower spine slightly forward. This position will feel "locked in place." Once you are in it you can meditate very deeply and the position will maintain itself. There are very few exercises or meditations which require this posture, but it is recognized as one of the best asanas for deep meditation.

Siddhasana or Perfect Pose

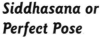

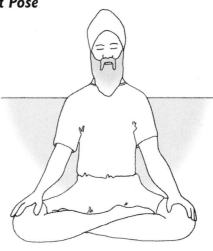

This posture is excellent for stimulating the nervous system and utilizing the body's sexual energy. It requires practice to perfect, but once it is mastered, simply sitting in this posture puts you into a meditative state.

Extend both legs straight. Bend the right leg and put the toes of the right foot in back of the left knee. Next bring the left heel under the right leg and under the sex organ. The left heel should touch the spot on the pelvis between the sex organ and the rectum. The toes of the right foot are contained in the bend of the left knee. Only the big toe is exposed. Pull the spine straight.

When you first begin to practice this asana do it for a few minutes only, building up gradually to as long as you like.

Vajrasana or Rock Pose

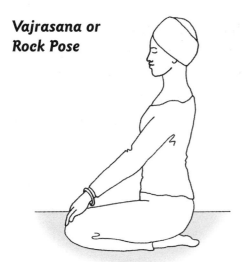

This asana is well known for its beneficial effects on the digestive system. It gained its nickname from the idea that one who masters this posture can sit in it and "digest rocks." It also makes you solid and balanced as a rock.

To get into the position, start by kneeling on both knees with the top of the feet on the ground. Sit back on the heels. The heels will press the two nerves that run into the lower center of each buttock. Keep the spine pulled straight.

Celibate Pose

A variation on Vajrasana, this pose requires a deep relaxation in the inner thigh and provides a very rooted, relaxed meditative seat. From Vajrasana, move the heels to the outside of the hips and allow the buttocks to relax down to the ground. The inner thighs roll inward and the tops of the feet are flat and point straight back, parallel to the hips. Ideally, the knees stay together. Allow the lower spine to press slightly forward, keeping the natural curve in the low back. The name implies its benefits; the practice of this asana balances the pelvis and the Second Chakra.

Virasana, Hero or Warrior Pose

Sit on the left heel, if possible placing the heel directly on the perineum, between the two sit bones. Bring

the right knee up toward the chest, placing the sole of the right foot on the ground. Hands come into Prayer Pose at the Heart Center.

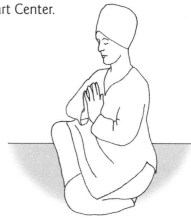

This pose is used during the Aquarian Sadhana's *Wahe Guru Wahe Guru Wahe Guru Wahe Jio* mantra. It generates a lot of heat in the body and a powerful magnetic field and expanded aura. It is the seat of the Warrior Saint.

Half Lotus

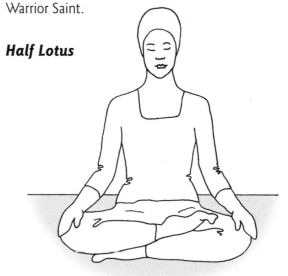

There are two poses frequently referred to as the Half Lotus position. The easier one is a variation of Sukasana. In Sukasana, pull the top foot all the way across onto the upper thigh instead of leaving it near the ankle.

The other Half Lotus is a little more difficult. Sit in Vajrasana and then stretch the right leg out straight. Bend the right leg so the foot rests on the upper left thigh. You are sitting and balancing on the left heel and the right knee. The pose is sometimes done with the legs switched when specifically indicated.

Sitting in a Chair

If none of these poses is comfortable for your meditation, you may sit in a chair—if you remember to choose the chair wisely. The tendency is to totally relax or slump in a chair. Be sure to counter this impulse by reminding yourself that you are sitting down to meditate—relaxed and totally attentive.

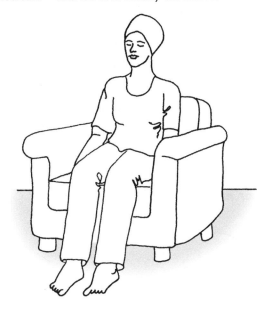

Pick a chair which gives you firm support. A large over-stuffed lounge chair may be uncomfortable for a long meditation. The back of the chair can give you support if it is straight. A common error is letting the legs hang loosely. It is essential that the feet be equally placed on the ground. The equal placement will assure that your lower spine and hips do not get out of balance.

Bound Lotus

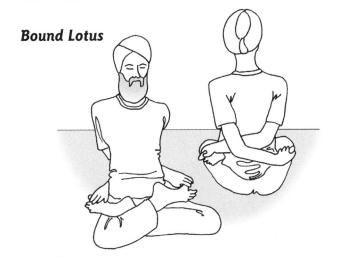

This posture is not as basic as the previous ones. It is difficult for many people. If you can do it, it is an excellent asana for deep meditation and glandular balancing. Get into the full lotus position. Push the feet as far up the thighs as possible. Reach around the back with both arms and grasp the big toes. The right hand grasps the toes of the right foot; the left hand grasps the left. Press the fleshy part of the big toes with the thumbs for pituitary stimulation. The spine is arched forward. The chin is held in. Do not force yourself into this position. Work slowly to gain the flexibility you need and begin to practice for a few minutes each day.

A variation of the posture can be achieved by relaxing the brow point down to the ground. This provides a deep healing for the nerves and the spine, but should be approached very cautiously and slowly. If you experience any pain in the knees or hips, come out of the posture and move more gradually toward this completed pose (using pillows or other props).

Thirty Degree Slant

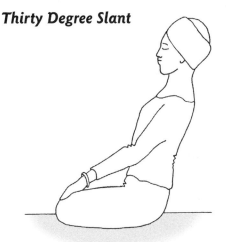

Sit in Easy Pose or Lotus Pose. Lean back 30° from vertical, keeping the spine straight. Don't slump back. Tilt the spine back. This will create a small pressure at the third and fourth lumbar vertebrae. The eyes are usually open slightly for meditation in this pose.

is magical as well as functional. Early in life we use our hands as our first exploration of the world and the things in it. We learn to grasp, let go, mold, shape, and create. The hand expresses our moods in each minute gesture. If you look at the palm you will see that the lines form intriguing patterns. If you understand the coding, the hands become an energy map of our consciousness and health. The yogis mapped out the hand areas and their associated reflexes. Each area of the hand reflexes to a certain area of the body or brain. Each area also represents different emotions or behaviors. By curling, crossing, stretching, and touching fingers to other fingers and areas of the palm, we can effectively talk to the body and mind. The hands become a keyboard for input in to our mind–body computer. Each mudra listed below is a technique for giving clear messages to the mind–body energy system.

Gyan Mudra

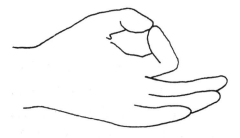

To form Gyan Mudra, put the tip of the thumb together with the tip of the index finger. This mudra stimulates knowledge and ability and gives you receptivity and calmness. The energy of the index finger is often symbolized by Jupiter, the planet representing expansion. The most commonly used mudra, it has two forms of practice: passive, as described above; and active. In the practice of powerful pranayams or exercises, the "active" form of the mudra is often used. In this case, the index finger is bent under the thumb so the fingernail is covered by the pad of the thumb and the three fingers remain straight and active.

Shuni Mudra

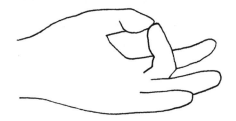

To form Shuni Mudra place the tip of the middle finger on the tip of the thumb. The three fingers remain straight. This mudra is said to give patience and discernment. The middle finger is often symbolized by the planet Saturn. Saturn represents the task master, the law of karma, the taking of responsibility and courage to hold to duty.

Surya or Ravi Mudra

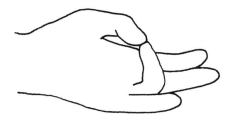

This mudra is formed by placing the tip of the ring finger on the tip of the thumb. The three fingers remain straight. Practicing it gives revitalizing energy, nerve strength, and good health. The quality of the ring finger is symbolized by the Sun or Uranus. The Sun represents energy, health, and sexuality. Uranus stands for nerve strength, intuition and change.

Buddhi Mudra

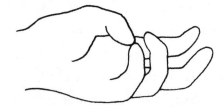

To form Buddhi Mudra place the tip of the little finger on the tip of the thumb. The three fingers remain straight. Practicing this opens the capacity to communicate clearly and intuitively. It also stimulates psychic development. The little finger is symbolized by Mercury for quickness and the mental powers of communication.

Venus Lock

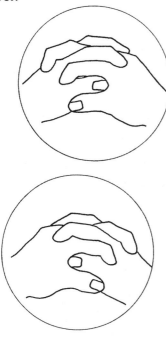

This mudra is used frequently in exercises. Its name is derived from the connection it creates between the positive and negative sides of the Venus mound on each hand and the thumbs. The thumbs represent the ego. The Venus mound is the fleshy area at the base of the thumb. It is symbolized by the planet Venus which is associated with the energy of sensuality and sexuality. The mudra channels the sexual energy and promotes glandular balance. It also brings the ability to focus or concentrate easily if you rest it in your lap while in a meditative posture. To form the mudra, place the palms facing each other. Interlace the fingers with the left little finger on the bottom. Put the left thumb tip on the webbing between the thumb and index finger of the right hand. The tip of the right thumb presses the fleshy mound at the base of the left thumb. Thumb positions are reversed for women and the right little finger goes on the bottom.

Prayer Mudra or Prayer Pose

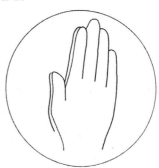

For this the palms of the hands are flat together. The positive side of the body (right, or masculine) and the negative side (left, or feminine) are neutralized. Generally this pose is placed at the Heart Center on the midline of the sternum and used to center yourself in preparation for doing a kriya, but is called for in other postures as well.

Bear Grip

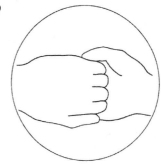

For Bear Grip place the left palm facing away from the chest and the right palm facing toward the chest. Bring the fingers together and curl them so that the hands form a single fist. Lock the position with the thumbs. This mudra is used to stimulate the heart and to intensify concentration.

Hands in the Lap

Another common mudra for meditation is formed by resting the right palm face-up in the lap with the left hand palm-up on top of it. Put the thumb tips together. The hand positions are reversed for men.

Mantras

Mantra has two fundamental meanings. The first is the mind's wave or projection. This implies that a mantra controls the waves of the mind through the use of sound. It is the most effective way to eliminate the flurry of thoughts released by the mind and suspend reactions to your subconscious projections. The second meaning is the resound or echo of the mind. This implies you listen to the sound and to the origin of the sound from the Infinite at the same time. You are consciously conscious of the sound and the echo or unstruck sound of that sound. This takes you past the surface of the sound and opens your intuitive capacity and neutral mind. Mantra is a technical device for regulating the mind. Mantras are discovered like gems in a mine or laws of energy in nature; they are not made up.

There are many mantras, each one has its own qualities, rhythm, and effects. The combined sound, resonance and rhythm of a mantra produce an altered state of consciousness which sets the pattern for the flow of thoughts. Mantra is not just an arbitrary label. It is a sound current which relates to its object. We always distinguish between a thing and its name because labels are arbitrary. Some languages make use of another level of sound. When a sound's innate vibration corresponds to or in some way reproduces what it refers to, it is a sacred language. This is the principle underlying languages such as Sanskrit and Gurmukhi. Chanting these ancient syllables is the fastest possible vibratory union between ourselves and the Creator. You determine which level of consciousness you want to relate to by the mantra you practice. The power of the mantra is decided by the level of consciousness you have. Mantra Yoga (or *Naad*) is the technique of yoking the individual with the whole. It is accomplished by merging the sound of the unit consciousness with the universal consciousness through the rhythmic power of the sound current (mantra).

Mantras projected toward Infinity relate to that frequency. If your total orientation and vibration is to make a lot of money, your words will reflect it. Chanting is the specialized use of one's vibratory capacities, taking the individual from his current position or level of development to his intended or projected destination. Mantra is the principle of reinforcement and rehearsal for the attainment of that ultimate destination.

In mantra, not only do we categorize the sounds according to their effects, but also according to their effectiveness and level from which they originate. *Bakri* refers to the sounds made at the tip of the tongue. It is audible sound, what you speak. *Khanth* is the sound generated at the throat. It is the sound of the mind, the thinking sounds. Practically speaking, it is the sound which one forms mentally when reading silently, where you hear the subvocal sound as though actually physically projected. *Hardhay* is the sound formed at the heart center. It is the communication generated from the heart. It is the wish the mother sends to her son or the *chela* (disciple) sends to the guru. It is a communion via the silent language of thought. *Nabhi* refers to the sound formed at the navel. What we speak at the navel is most powerful. The last category is *Anahat*, the sound which has no end, infinite. It is the "unstruck sound," which reverberates deep into all levels of consciousness and existence.

In the deepest meditation when the mind and body merge in union with the spirit essence, *Anahat* is the sound that is heard. This vibratory frequency is actually heard in children and its highest conscious development occurs around the age of one and a half years. In modern society, with all the cluttering of our consciousness that industrialized society produces, this sound, which should otherwise be easily and regularly experienced, gradually loses its prominence in the mind and is usually unheard and forgotten by the age of three. It is through the practice of mantra and the remembrance of the name and sound of creative Infinity that one may revitalize and redevelop that lost experience of the *Anahat*, the unstruck melody.

All these levels of sound are developed and integrated in a good sadhana over a long period of time. Ultimately the practice of mantra is perfected so that all mantra is *japa*. *Ja* means sound, *pa* means resound. *Japa* means "to resound the mantra." In *japa* the mantra is projected to the infinite cosmos and reflected back to you. You can hear it without feeling you produced it. It is the experience of a million voices echoing the mantra. It is cozy and creative. This *japa* leads to *tapa*, the inner psychic heat of *prana*. It is *tapa* that cleans and strengthens the nerves. The practice of *japa* is often done with the aid of a string of beads known as a mala. A mala is designed with a calculated number of beads (usually 108, 54 or 27). On each bead the mantra or meditation is repeated. In addition, there is a "guru bead" or *meru*, which is slightly larger than the rest and reminds the practitioner that she has completed one full cycle of the mala. The guru bead is not crossed, one merely turns the mala and returns in the opposite direction. Originally the mala was used to measure the length of time of the meditation practiced. Instead of doing a meditation for, say, thirty-one minutes, one might do "25 malas." In addition, the necessity of changing direction every 108 repetitions helps to maintain alertness in the practitioner, which by nature declines after many repetitions of the same mental sequence.

The mala also seems to provide a source of stimulation for the nervous system and brain through the continuous pressing of the fingertips on the beads. In all chants it is important to move the mouth and enunciate; recite, not just speak. There is a tendency to mumble, slur, or project the sound without moving the lips and tongue. The total effect of mantra depends on the reflex points on the tongue and in the mouth. So enunciate and move the tongue precisely.

Types of Mantra

There are two types of mantras frequently used in Kundalini Yoga. The first is the *bij* mantra, which is like a seed. It is the name of God planted inside of you, in your heart, where it will grow and spread its radiance throughout your aura. But before the seed can be planted, the soil must be prepared. And for that we use an *ashtang* mantra. *Ashtang* means "eight-fold." Just as the spermatozoa must circle the egg eight times before penetrating, so too must the *bij* mantra be implanted in the heart within the eight-fold vibration of the *ashtang* mantra. The eight-fold vibration acts as a stimulant that balances the entire brain. It is only an *ashtang* mantra or the *Panj Shabd* mantra that can provide this total stimulation of your potential. What follows are various commonly used mantras in the practice of Kundalini Yoga, representing either the *bij* or *ashtang* sound currents.

Adi Shakti Mantra (or Morning Call):
Ek Ong Kaar Sat Naam Siree Wha-hay Guroo

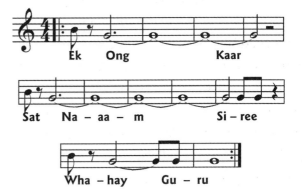

There are many ashtang mantras, but one that we chant most regularly is called the Adi Shakti Mantra. There are two ways to experience and find the Divine. One is to open the solar plexus and charge your solar centers so that you get directly connected. The other is to concentrate and meditate and experience the sound of *shabd* within your solar centers from the crown chakra and receive the divine light. This mantra incorporates both methods.

The mantra is very precise; the sounds are exact keys which you touch to telegraph your message to the Infinite Self. Your entire system is played by these sounds. Each sound vibrates and integrates a different chakra to its full radiance within the aura. *Ek* means one. It is the essence of all which is one. *Ong,* as stated above, is the primal vibration from which all creativity flows. You go beyond all limiting conceptions of the world, and self, and penetrate to the creative core that supports it all through the sound of *Ong.* The sound is created in the upper palate and nose. It vibrates the entire skull and has a full nasal tone. *Kar* means creation or actions in the creation. *Sat* means truth; *Nam* means name, or, as Yogi Bhajan often spoke of it, identity. The name of the One Creator known through creation is not a word, but truth- reality and existence itself. When you chant *Sat,* briefly contract the navel and lower centers to release some of the inner power of creation. *Siri* means great. *Wha* is the untranslatable expression of experiencing the Creator's supreme power. It is ecstasy. *He* is now or that it is. *Wahe* means the infinite ecstasy beyond thought that is. *Guru* means wisdom, that which brings you from darkness to light. Together, one can translate it as: "There exists one Creator throughout the creation whose name is truth. Great is the ecstasy of being brought from darkness to light."

The mantra may be divided into three parts. *Ek Ong Kar* means, "There is one Creator who has created this creation." Here you realize the need for a conscious union with the Infinite. *Sat Nam* means "Truth is His Name." It says the *Nam* or form of identity is *Sat* or all that exists. *Sat Nam* is the name of God that we relate to; it is the *bij* mantra, the seed that we are planting in our hearts. With *Sat Nam,* we pierce to the core of truth and understand the nature of reality. The third part of the Adi Shakti Mantra is *Siri Wahe Guru.* It means "great, indescribable beyond words is His wisdom." Here you express the bliss of truly knowing yourself. As Yogi Bhajan has said, "If you chant this mantra during these dark ages of the Kali Yug, it will open the lock of ignorance and darkness. This will liberate you and unite you with the Divine. In the period of two and one-half hours before the rising of the sun, when the channels are most clear, if the mantra is sung in sweet harmony, you will be one with the Lord. This will open your solar plexus, which in turn will charge the solar center. The solar complex will get connected with the cosmic energy and you will be liberated from the cycles of karma that bind you to this Earth. All mantras are good because they all awaken the divine, but this mantra is the mantra for this time. It represents the path of progressive spiritual knowledge of the self."

Chanting this mantra means unlimited attachment to the Infinite beyond any man or finite form. Those who attach themselves to a man or personality end up miserable. Yogi Bhajan says, "It is equal to millions and billions of suns. When you recite this mantra, the day shall come when you shall have the light within you. You will find it equal to you cannot say what. There is no vocabulary and there is no tongue which can say just how bright that light is. But remember that light; you shall see that it is the only light through which you can overcome the cycle of karma. Then nothing disturbs you. Then you live normally, and you are beyond the power of the cycles of time and space." There is no need for secret mantras and all the gimmickry so often resorted to. This mantra is open to all—without initiations and cults—yet it is basic to the awakening and regulating of the kundalini energy: the basic evolutionary force in the total human psyche.

This mantra may be chanted in the two and one-half breath cycle for its full power, or in any tune you make up for light meditation. In the two and one-half breath cycle, you take a deep inhale and chant *Ek Ong Kar* in one breath. The *Ek* is very short, *Ong* and *Kar* are long but equal in length. Take another deep inhale and chant *Sat Nam Siri*. The *Sat* is short, *Nam* is very long (should be the same interval as *Ong* and *Kar* together), and *Siri* just escapes your tongue with the last bit of breath as you lift the diaphragm slightly. Then take a short half breath and chant *Wahe Guru*. *Wha* is short and *Hay Guru* is longer but short relative to the first two phrases.

Sat Nam
Sa—a—a—at Nam

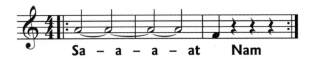

Sat Nam is the *bij*, or seed mantra that is most used in the practice of Kundalini Yoga. It is a universal mantra which is not limited to Kundalini Yoga. It represents the sound embodiment of Truth itself.

Sat (truth), the reality of what exists; *Nam* (name, identity), the vibration which creates what it names. When *Sat Nam* is chanted in its *bij* form, it is usually chanted in a breath ratio of 8 to 1, 26 to 1 or 35 to 1. That is, the time of *Sat* is 8, 26, or 35 times that of *Nam*. This mantra can be used to smooth out and balance mental energy. It gives you a feeling of reality. It can also be used to release energy.

As you chant this mantra extend your mind to Infinity and remember that "in the beginning there was the Word, and the Word was God."

This God, this Word, lives inside of you. You are a manifestation of that. Tune into that Infinity. Project a call from your heart. The Infinity that created you is not deaf; and does not live very far away. The power of mantra is the power of manifestation. If we recite the mantra from complete innocence, it will take the mind and heart to an experience of its origin in the Creator.

Ashtang Bij Mantra
Sat Nam Sat Nam Sat Nam Sat Nam
Sat Nam Sat Nam Wahe Guru

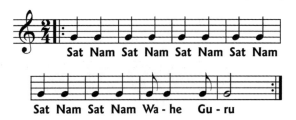

This is an *ashtang* mantra that uses only *bij* mantras as syllables. One of the most potent and frequently used mantras is *Sat Nam, Sat Nam, Sat Nam, Sat Nam, Sat Nam, Sat Nam, Wahe Guru*. This mantra works the tongue. Your throat will get dry at first until you master the rhythm. It can generate the power of creative sound in your words. Each *Sat Nam* is one count in the rhythm. *Wahe Guru* is two counts. One repetition takes about 3 to 4 seconds. To keep the rhythm there is a slight inhale on a half-count between repetitions.

Panj Shabd: Sa Ta Na Ma

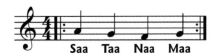

This is the nuclear form of the *bij* mantra, *Sat Nam*. Here each syllable of sound is created in a ratio to the other. Adding this melody and rhythm makes the mantra a form of Laya Yoga. *Panj* means five; the five primal sounds are SA-TA-NA-MA. SA means Infinity; TA, life; NA, death; and MA, birth or resurrection. The fifth sound is the common A which means to come. These five sounds are known as the Panj Shabd.

Guru Gaitri Mantra:
Gobinday, Mukanday, Udaaray, Apaaray,
Hareerung, Kareeung, Nirnaamay, Akaamy

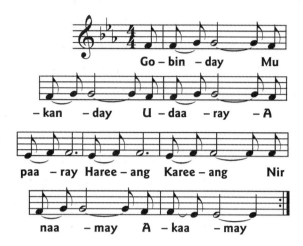

This mantra has a very special quality—it eliminates karmic blocks and curses from the past and cleanses the aura so that it becomes easier to meditate and relate to the Infinite. It was given by Guru Gobind Singh and is found in the Tenth Guru's work, *Jaap Sahib*. It is also an *ashtang* mantra with eight major components. If this mantra is practiced regularly for 31 minutes to 2½ hours daily, it will cause all the occult powers to serve you. The mantra translates: "Sustainer, Liberator, Enlightener, Infinite, Destroyer, Creator, Nameless, Desireless." These are eight aspects or names of the Godhead. The mantra cleanses the subconscious and produces the Shakti sun energy in every nerve. If a person is too mentally and physically blocked to let the vibratory effect of the Adi Shakti Mantra take hold, this mantra will clear the way. It is chanted in the above musical notation, with one full cycle per breath.

Guru Mantra:
Guroo guroo wha-hay guroo
guroo ram das guroo

This mantra relates directly to healing and protective energy represented by Guru Ram Das, the Fourth Guru of the Sikhs. He is held in reverence by all people who respect universal service. It is by the grace of the house

of Guru Ram Das that through his humble servant, Yogi Bhajan, the veils of secrecy have been lifted from the teachings of Kundalini Yoga. This mantra is an *ashtang* mantra. It was given to the Yogi Bhajan from a deep meditation on Guru Ram Das, his guru on the etheric plane. It is comprised of two parts. The first part is a *nirgun* mantra (Guru Guru Wahe Guru). The second part is a *sirgun* mantra (Guru Ram Das Guru). *Nirgun* means without quality. A *nirgun* mantra is one which has no finite components and vibrates only to Infinity. A *sirgun* mantra is one which represents form. This Guru Mantra projects the mind to Infinity, then allows a finite, guiding relationship to come into your awareness and activities. The first part of the mantra, *Guru Guru Wahe Guru*, projects the mind to the source of knowledge and ecstasy. The second part, *Guru Ram Das Guru*, means "the wisdom that comes as a servant of the Infinite." It is the mantra of humility. It reconnects the experience of infinity to the finite.

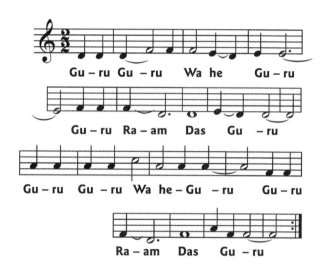

The mantra is chanted a number of ways: the most common one is given in musical notation above. Try to chant complete cycles of the mantra with each breath. It will give you relaxation, self-healing and emotional relief.

Wahe Guru: A Mantra of Ecstasy
Wha-hay Guroo Wha-hay Guroo
Wha-hay Wha-hay Wha-hay Guroo

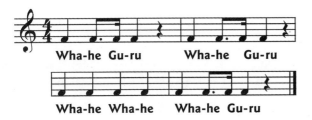

The *bij* mantra, *Wahe Guru*, done in an *ashtang* form is *Wahe Guru, Wahe Guru, Wahe, Wahe, Wahe Guru*. It is a mantra that produces a sense of happiness. It is often used in kriyas that develop healing abilities. It has a rhythm that is the Laya Yoga form so it easily stays with the subconscious with minimal practice.

Laya Yoga Kundalini Mantra: Adi Shakti
Ek Ong Kaar-(uh)
Sat-a Naam-(uh)
Siree Wha-(uh) Hay Guroo

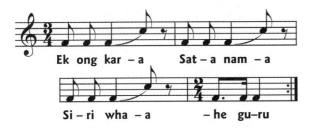

This is the Laya Yoga form of the Adi Shakti Mantra, which is very powerful and can suspend the mind into a kind of blissful trance of connectedness. The mantra is changed slightly by adding the "uh" sound to the three primary sections of the mantra, giving it rhythm and additional power: Ek Ong Kaar-(uh), Sat-a Naam-(uh), Siree Wha-(uh) Hay Guru. The rhythm of the chant gives it a sense of "spinning." It rotates the energy of all the chakras and the aura.

The navel point is pulled in sharply on *Ek*. With each "uh," the diaphragm is pulled up so that the rib cage lifts. On *Hay Guroo*, the stomach and diaphragm relax.

As you chant, visualize the energy spinning from the base of the spine upward through the top of the head to Infinity. On *Ek* see the energy start from the navel point and go downward. On the first "uh," the energy pierces the First Chakra at the base of the spine. On the second "uh," it coils through the lock on the spine at the level of the diaphragm and heart center. On the third "uh," you spin the energy past the neck and throat chakra. On *Hay Guroo* let the energy go through the top of the skull, the Seventh Chakra, into infinity. If you get into the rhythm of the spin, the breath will automatically ebb in and out at 3½ cycles per chant. The spine will heat up and sweat. It is a mantra of total absorption into Infinity.

There are many other mantras, but this collection has most of the basic chants needed for an excellent beginning to the practice of Kundalini Yoga.

Bandhas

Bandhas or locks are used frequently in Kundalini Yoga. Combinations of muscle contractions, each lock has the function of changing blood circulation, nerve pressure, and the flow of cerebral spinal fluid. They also direct the flow of psychic energy, *prana*, into the main energy channels that relate to raising the kundalini energy. They concentrate the body's energy for use in consciousness and self-healing. There are three important locks: *jalandhar bandh*, *uddiyana bandh*, and *mulbandh*. When all three locks are applied simultaneously, it is called *mahabandh*, the Great Lock.

Jalandhar Bandh or Neck Lock

The most basic lock used in Kundalini Yoga is *jalandhar bandh*, the Neck Lock. This lock is practiced by gently stretching the back of the neck straight and pulling the ching toward the back of the neck. Lift the chest and sternum and keep the muscles of the neck and throat and face relaxed. The head stays level without tilting the chin down or forward. The spinal vertebrae in the neck straighten to allow the increased flow of pranic energy to travel freely into the upper glandular centers of the brain. This is critical. In Kundalini Yoga kriyas, a vast energy is generated that produces psychic heat which opens the pranic *nadis* (channels) that may be blocked. When this opening happens, there can sometimes be a quick shift in blood pressure causing dizziness. *Jalandhar bandh* regulates this phenomenon.

By applying this lock, the thyroid and parathyroid glands are stimulated which causes them to secrete optimally and activate the higher functions of the pituitary. If the lock is not applied, the breathing exercises can cause uncomfortable pressure in the eyes, ears, and hearing. It is a general rule to apply *jalandhar bandh* in all meditations unless otherwise specified.

Uddiyana Bandh or Diaphragm Lock

Applied by lifting the diaphragm up high into the thorax and pulling the upper abdominal muscles back toward the spine, *uddiyana bandh* gently massages the intestines and the heart muscle. The spine should be straight and it is most often applied on the exhale. Applied forcefully on the inhale, it can create pressure in the eyes and the heart.

It is considered a powerful lock because it allows the pranic force to move through the central nerve channel of the spine penetrating the neck region. It also has a direct link to stimulating the hypothalamic–pituitary–adrenal axis in the brain. It stimulates the sense of compassion and can give a new youthfulness to the entire body. In Laya Yoga Kundalini Mantra, the rhythmic application of this lock is crucial to attaining the highest effects of the chanting.

Mulbandh or Root Lock

The Root Lock is the most commonly applied lock but also the most complex. It coordinates and combines the energy of the rectum, sex organs, and navel point. Mul is the root, base, or source. The first part of the *mulbandh* is to contract the anal sphincter and draw it in and up as if trying to hold back a bowel movement. Then draw up the sex organ so the urethral tract is contracted. Finally, pull in the navel point by drawing back the lower abdomen towards the spine so the rectum and sex organs are drawn up toward the navel point. This action unites the two major energy flows of the body: *prana* and *apana*. Prana is the positive, generative energy of the upper body and heart center. *Apana* is the downward flow of eliminating energy. *Mulbandh* pulls the *apana* up and the *prana* down to the navel point. This combination of energies generates the necessary psychic heat to release the kundalini energy. This lock is applied on the exhale. It can also be applied on the inhale when specified.

Mahabandh or The Great Lock

This is the application of all three locks simultaneously. When all the locks are applied, the nerves and glands are rejuvenated. The practice and perfection of *mahabandh* is said to relieve wet dreams and preoccupation with sexual fantasy. It regulates blood pressure, reduces menstrual cramping, and puts extra blood circulation into the lower glands: testes, ovaries, prostate, etc.

Pranayam is the science of controlling and conserving prana through breath techniques which change the physical, mental, and energetic states of our lives.

Who among you has the power to breathe?

What is breath to you?

It means life.

It is life.

What is life?

Life is a bindu, a point.

Life is not under your control and the mind is not obedient, but there is something the mind does obey. That is the rate of the breath. . . . When the breath is long and deep and slow, the mind is constant and one-pointed. . . . If you can train yourself to breathe eight breaths per minute, you can have your temper and your projection under control. It is the most creative meditation you can do.

Sitali Pranayam

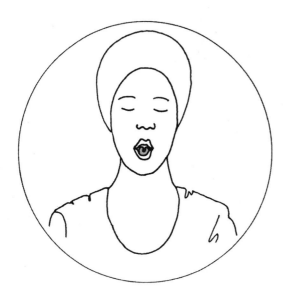

Sit in a comfortable meditative posture with the spine straight. Curl the tongue and protrude it slightly past the lips. Inhale deeply and smoothly over the tongue. Exhale through the nose. Continue for **5 minutes**. Then inhale—hold. Pull in the tongue. Exhale and relax. **Repeat this for two more 5-minute periods**.

Comments:

Sitali Pranayam is a well-known practice. It soothes and cools you. It gives you robust sexual and digestive energy. This breath is often used for lowering fever. Great powers of rejuvenation and detoxification are attributed to this breath when practiced regularly. Doing 52 breaths daily can even extend your vitality throughout your lifespan. It is practiced for varying lengths of time within many kriyas and is practiced by itself as a health giving pranayam. Often the tongue may taste bitter at first. This is a sign of natural detoxification. As you continue the practice, the taste of the tongue will become sweet.

1. Sit in Easy Pose. Extend the arms straight up, hugging the ears, with the palms together. Begin **Breath of Fire** and continue for **2 minutes**. Inhale—hold for 20 seconds, exhale. **Repeat Breath of Fire** for **2 minutes**. Inhale—hold 30 seconds, exhale. Repeat one more time. Relax for 2 minutes.

2. Sit on the heels in Vajrasana or Rock Pose. Cross the arms behind the head and hold onto the shoulders. Begin **Breath of Fire** and continue for **2 minutes.** Inhale—hold. Exhale—relax. **Repeat Breath of Fire** for **1 minute**. Relax for 3 minutes.

3. Yoga Mudra: Sit on the heels. Place the hands in Venus Lock behind the back and lean forward, bringing the forehead to the ground. Raise the arms straight up to 90°, maintaining the position to your maximum ability. Hold for at least **3 minutes**.

4. Relax completely on the back for 10 minutes.

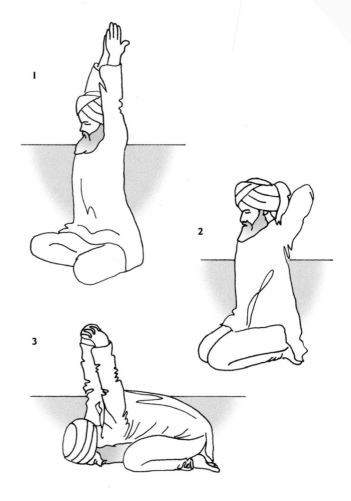

Comments:

The skin breathes. It is just as important to keep its channels clean as it is for the nose or the lungs. This series removes obstructions to the flow of *prana* through this third "lung"—the skin.

Pranayam for Purification

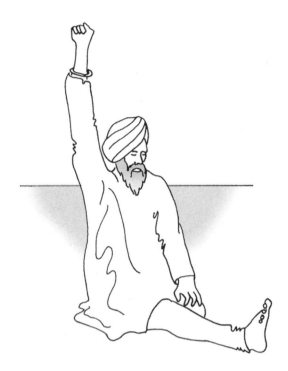

Sit on the left heel with the right leg extended forward. Stretch the right arm straight up and make a fist. Take long deep breaths through the right nostril. **Mentally vibrate *Sat*** with the inhale and ***Nam*** with the exhale. Continue for **3 minutes**. Then switch legs, arms, and nostrils. **Continue for 3 minutes**. The more you stretch the arm, the more the corresponding nostril will open.

Comments:

This breathing kriya is to eliminate negativity and the urge to slander others rather than purify yourself. It stimulates the lymphatic system to cleanse itself. It increases strength and responsiveness of the nervous system throughout the body.

Kriya for Expanding Lung Capacity

1. Sit in **Easy Pose**. Raise the arms up with the elbows bent at a right angle. Now bend the wrists so that the palms are facing up. Maintain this position for **1 minute**. To end: Inhale deeply and hold for 10 seconds. Exhale. Repeat 3 more times then exhale and hold the breath out. Apply *mulbandh*. Inhale, hold briefly and exhale.

2. Sit in **Easy Pose** with **Venus Lock** in the lap. Begin **Long Deep Breathing for 10 minutes**. With each inhalation, fully expand and raise the rib cage. If you are not used to breathing in this full, deep, smooth manner, you might experience a transient adjustment or get light headed. Though an infrequent effect, it passes quickly if it occurs. Firm concentration at the brow will alleviate most imbalances. If it persists, stop and be sure your breathing pattern is correct and that you are not paradoxically breathing. If you are a beginner, you can breathe for a shorter time, stop briefly, and resume the practice until the time is completed. Very quickly you will be able to do the entire time comfortably and with increasing steadiness, alertness and vitality. Move from this exercise immediately into the next.

3. Sit up with the legs extended. Bend forward and hold the toes. Inhale; exhale and hold the breath out. Pump the belly as long as possible, then inhale and exhale; repeat 2 more times.

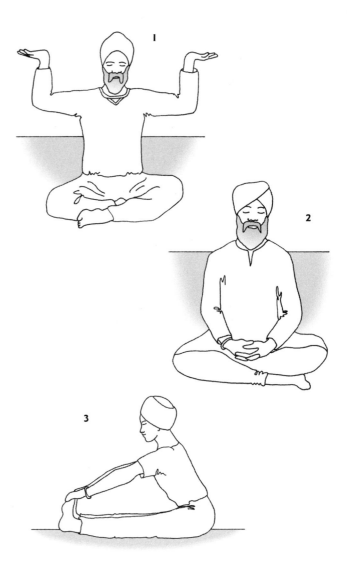

Comments:

Exercise 1 turns on the energy to the lungs and heart. Exercise 2 uses the energy to expand the lung capacity. Exercise 3 balances and distributes the *prana*. For a beginners' class, do this set 3 times, but allow only 2 or 3 minutes of breathing in Exercise 2.

Basic Breath Series

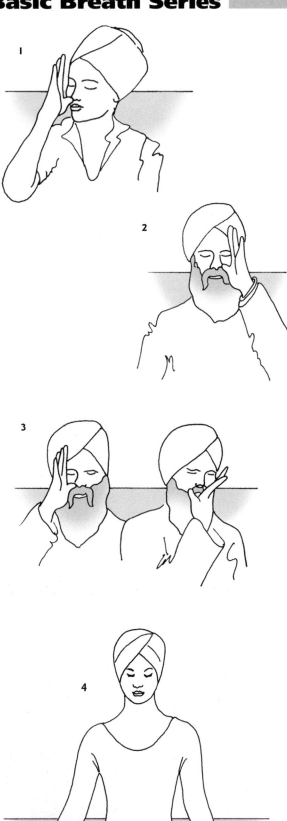

1. Sit in **Easy Pose**. Block the right nostril with the thumb and make an antenna of the right-hand fingers. Begin **Long Deep Breathing** through the left nostril for **3 minutes**. Inhale—hold for 10 seconds.

2. Repeat the first exercise on the left side, using the left thumb to block the left nostril. Continue for 3 minutes. Inhale—hold for 10 seconds.

3. **Inhale** through the **left nostril**, **exhale** through the **right** using Long Deep Breathing. Use the thumb and little finger to close alternate nostrils. Continue **3 minutes**. Now **reverse** the alternate nostril breath for **3 more minutes**; inhale through the right and exhale through the left.

4. Sit in **Easy Pose** with hands in **Gyan Mudra**. Begin **Breath of Fire**. Center yourself at the Brow Point. Continue with a regular powerful breath for **7¹/₂ minutes**. Then inhale, suspend the breath, circulating the energy. Exhale and relax or meditate for 5 minutes.

5. Sit in a meditative pose. **Chant** long *Sat Nam*. Continue **3–15 minutes**. End with a deep inhale, relax the breath and be still for several moments.

Comments:

This set opens the *pranic* channels and balances the breath in the two sides of your body. It is often practiced before a more strenuous, physical *kriya*. It is great to do on its own whenever you need a quick lift and a clear mind.

Pranayam Series 1

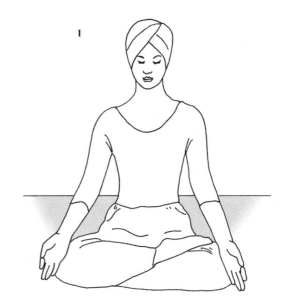

1. Sit in **Easy Pose** with the hands in **Gyan Mudra** and the arms straight. Begin **Breath of Fire** and continue for **7 minutes**. Inhale—hold the breath for 30 seconds, exhale.

2. Begin **Long Deep Breathing** through both nostrils. Breathe deeper than normal so that the entire rib cage lifts and expands several inches. Continue **5 minutes**, then inhale—hold 15 seconds, exhale.

3. Immediately begin to **inhale** through **puckered lips** and **exhale** through the **nose**. Continue **3 minutes**. Then inhale—hold briefly, exhale.

4. Do a powerful and regular **Breath of Fire** for **2 minutes**. Then inhale deeply—hold as long as is comfortable. Focus at the Brow Point.

5. Meditate with normal breathing. Feel the flow of energy through the whole body.

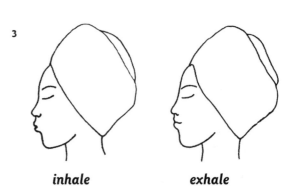

inhale   *exhale*

Pranayam Series 2

Sit in Easy Pose with the left hand in Gyan Mudra and block the right nostril with the right thumb. Inhale through the left nostril; block the left nostril with the little finger and exhale through the right nostril. Think *Sat* on the inhale and *Nam* on the exhale. Continue for 10 minutes with deep, regular breaths. Then inhale, exhale, and inhale, exhale completely and holding the breath out, apply *mulbandh*. Inhale and relax.

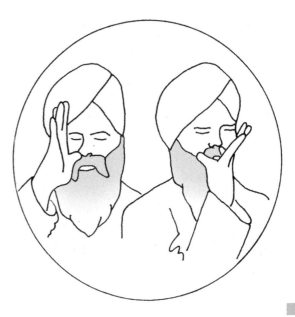

Comments:

The first kriya is a good blood cleanser and energizer. The second is for emotional balance. If some morning you feel that you "got up on the wrong side of bed," this exercise will rebalance you for the day.

Ungali Pranayam

Sit with a straight spine. Meditate on the sound. Inhale, exhale and **then** begin a segmented breath on the sound—15 breaks on both the inhale and the exhale.

For example:
Inhale: SA SA SA SA . . .15 "sniffs" or segments of breath
Exhale: TA TA TA TA . . .
Inhale: NA NA NA NA . . .
Exhale: MA MA MA MA . . .

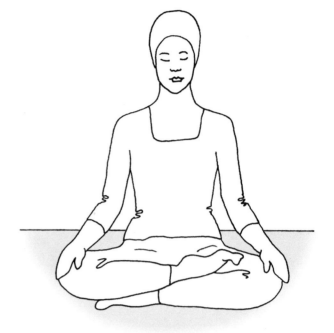

Comments:

Start with **3 minutes**. Each time you practice, add 1 minute, working up to 31 minutes. In order to concentrate on the mantra, **Sa Ta Na Ma**, use a mala or your hand to count to 15 and allow the mind to rest in the sound current. Yogi Bhajan points out that first we must master *Sa Ta Na Ma*; then *Wahe Guru* will aid in our journey to reach our destiny. This pranayam can cause dizziness so Yogi Bhajan emphasized **the necessity to have someone stand by you in case you faint**. It activates the central brain—the pituitary, pineal and frontal areas; coordinates the individual functioning of the 10 regions of the left and right brains; and when accompanied by appropriate greens in the diet it will help reduce weight.

A kriya is a technique used in Kundalini Yoga to produce an altered state of consciousness. This technique can be a meditation or an exercise or both. Every exercise is not a kriya. By doing a kriya, a sequence of physical and mental events is initiated that affect the body, mind and spirit. Each kriya makes a specific claim as to its effects, but all balance the chakras, stimulate the glandular system, and strengthen the nervous system.

In this section you will find kriyas of varying difficulty. Some, such as Sat Kriya, are single exercise meditations, while others are exercise sets with multiple postures followed by a meditation or relaxation. Accompanying each kriya is a commentary on the physical, mental, and/or spiritual effects produced by practicing it. When a kriya is mastered, the practitioner gains easy and immediate access to a particular state of emotion or consciousness.

All of the kriyas, as well as the information included in the sections on basics and meditation, are directly from the teachings of Yogi Bhajan, Master of Kundalini Yoga, the Yoga of Awareness.

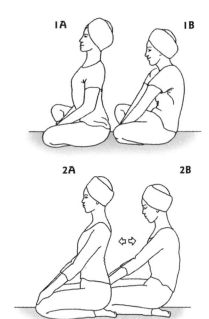

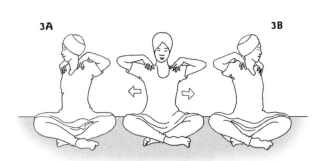

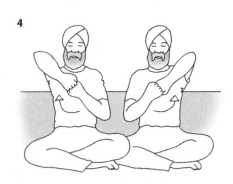

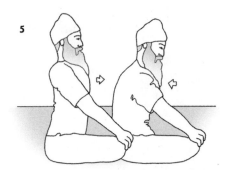

1. Sit in **Easy Pose**. Grab the ankles or shins with both hands and deeply inhale as you flex the spine forward and lift the chest up. On the exhale, flex the spine back. Keep the head level so it does not flip-flop. Repeat **108 times**. To end: Inhale center and exhale relax. Rest 1 Minute.

2. Sit in *Vajrasana*, on the heels. Place the hands flat on the thighs. Continue spine flex in this position. Inhaling as the spine flexes forward, exhaling back. Mentally vibrate *Sat* on the inhale, *Nam* on the exhale. Repeat **108 times**. Rest 2 minutes.

3. Sit in Easy Pose and grasp the shoulders, with fingers in front, thumbs in back. **Inhale** and twist to the **left**, **exhale** and twist to the **right**. Breathing is long and deep. Continue **26 times**. To end: Inhale center; exhale relax. Rest 1 minute.

4. Lock the fingers in **Bear Grip** at the Heart Center. Move the elbows in a see-saw motion, breathing deeply with the motion at about one see saw per second. Continue **26-108 times**; then inhale, exhale, and pull, as if trying to pull the hands apart. Relax 30 seconds.

5. Still in Easy Pose, grasp the knees firmly and, **keeping the elbows straight**, begin to flex the upper spine. Inhale forward, exhale back. Repeat **108 times**. Rest 1 minute.

Comments:

Age is measured by the flexibility of the spine; to stay young, stay flexible. This series works systematically from the base of the spine to the top. All 26 vertebrae receive stimulation and all the chakras receive a burst of energy. It is a good series to do before meditation or as a warm-up before a more strenuous kriya.

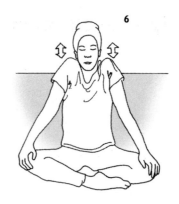

6. **Shoulder Shrug**: Bring both shoulders up toward the ears with the inhale and relax down with the exhale. Do this for **less than** 2 minutes at a pace of about 12 shrugs per 10 seconds. Inhale and hold 15 seconds with shoulders pressed up. Relax.

7. **Roll the neck** slowly to the right **five times**, then to the left **five times**. To end: Inhale the head to the center.

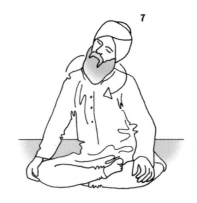

8. Lock the fingers in **Bear Grip at the throat**. Inhale—apply *mulbandh*; exhale—apply *mulbandh*. Then raise the hands above the top of the head. Inhale—apply *mulbandh*. Exhale—apply *mulbandh*. Repeat the entire cycle two more times.

9. **Sat Kriya**: Sit on the heels and stretch the arms overhead so that the elbows hug the ears. With the palms together, interlock all the fingers except the index fingers (Jupiter) which point straight up. Men cross the right thumb over the left with the left little finger on the bottom; women cross left thumb over right, right pinkie on bottom. Begin to chant *Sat Nam* emphatically in a constant rhythm about 8 times per 10 seconds. Chant *Sat* from the Navel Point and solar plexus, pulling the umbilicus all the way in toward the spine. On *Nam* relax the belly. Continue at least **3 minutes**, then inhale and squeeze the muscles tightly from the buttocks all the way up the back, past the shoulders. Mentally allow the energy to flow through the top of the skull.

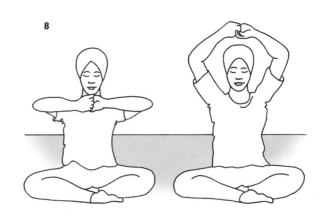

10. Relax completely on your back for 15 minutes.

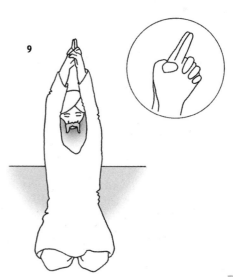

In a beginner's class, each exercise that lists 108 repetitions can be done 26 times. The rest periods are then extended as appropriate.

Many people report greater mental clarity and alacrity after regular practice of this kriya. A contributing factor is the increased circulation of the spinal fluid, which is crucially linked to having a good memory.

Sat Kriya

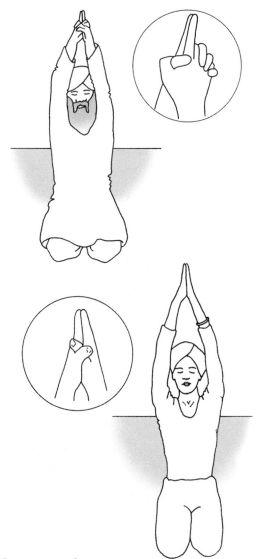

Sit on the heels and stretch the arms overhead so that the elbows hug the ears. With the palms together, interlock all the fingers except the index fingers (Jupiter) which point straight up. Men cross the right thumb over the left with the left little finger on the bottom; women cross left thumb over right, right pinkie on bottom. Begin to chant **Sat Nam** emphatically in a constant rhythm about 8 times per 10 seconds. Chant the sound **Sat** from the Navel Point and solar plexus, pulling the umbilicus all the way in toward the spine. On **Nam** relax the belly.

Continue at least **3 minutes**, then inhale and squeeze the muscles tightly from the buttocks all the way up the back, past the shoulders. Mentally allow the energy to flow through the top of the skull. Ideally, you should **relax for twice the length of time that the kriya was practiced**.

Comments:

Sat Kriya is fundamental to Kundalini Yoga and should be practiced every day for at least 3 minutes. If you have time for nothing else, make this kriya part of your daily commitment to yourself to keep the body a clean and vital temple of God.

Notice that you emphasize pulling the Navel Point in. Don't try to apply *mulbandh*; it happens automatically if the navel is pulled. Consequently, the hips and lumbar spine do not rotate or flex. Your spine stays straight and the only motion your arms make is a slight up-and-down stretch with each **Sat Nam** as your chest lifts.

Sat Kriya's effects are numerous. It strengthens the entire sexual system and stimulates its natural flow of energy, relaxing phobias about sexuality. It allows you to control the insistent sexual impulse by redirecting the flow of sexual energy to creative activities and healing in the body. People who are severely maladjusted or who have mental problems benefit from this kriya because these disturbances are always connected with an imbalance in the energies of the lower three chakras. General physical health is improved because all of the internal organs receive a gentle, rhythmic massage from this exercise. The heart gets stronger from the rhythmic up-and-down of blood pressure you generate from the pumping motion of the navel. This exercise works directly on stimulating and channeling the kundalini energy, so it must always be practiced with the mantra *Sat Nam*. You may build the time of the kriya to 31 minutes, but remember to have a long, deep relaxation immediately afterwards. A good way to build the time up is to do the kriya for 3 minutes, then rest 2 minutes. Repeat this cycle until you have completed 15 minutes of Sat Kriya and 10 minutes of rest. Then follow this sequence with an additional 15–20 minutes of deep relaxation. Do not try to jump to 31 minutes because you feel you are strong, virile or happen to be a yoga teacher. Respect the inherent power of the technique. Let the kriya prepare the ground of your body properly to plant the seed of higher experience. It is not just an exercise, it is a kriya that works on all levels of your being—known and unknown. You might block the more subtle experiences of higher energies by pushing the physical body too hard. You could have a huge rush of energy or you may have an experience of higher consciousness, but then not be able to integrate the experience into your psyche. So prepare yourself with constancy, patience and moderation. The end result is assured.

If you have not taken drugs or have cleared your system of all their effects, you may choose to practice this kriya with the palms open, pressing flat against each other. This releases more energy than the other method. It is generally not taught this way in a public class because someone attending may have totally weakened his nerves through drug abuse.

Sit straight in a cross-legged position. Raise the right arm straight up, lifting the shoulder, with the palm facing toward you, fingers spread wide. The left hand rests on the left knee. Eyes are closed. Chant *Sat Nam* in a constant rhythm, about 8 times per 10 seconds. Chant **Sat** from the navel, pulling the Navel Point all the way in toward the spine. On **Nam**, relax the belly. Continue for 11, 22 or 31 minutes. To end: Inhale, hold and squeeze the entire body, bringing the energy up. Exhale and relax.

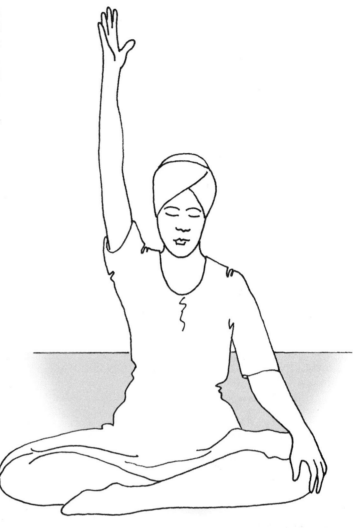

Comments:

"Give yourself values. Character will only come when your body, mind and soul are committed to you. This body will become diseased and it will go. In between you have to emit light so you can leave behind a legacy. If you understand this you will not do countless nonsense. You are made of God. You are part of God. Change your angle, from being physical and mental, to be angelic." A daily practice of Sat Kriya is the essence of life.

Kriya For Morning Sadhana

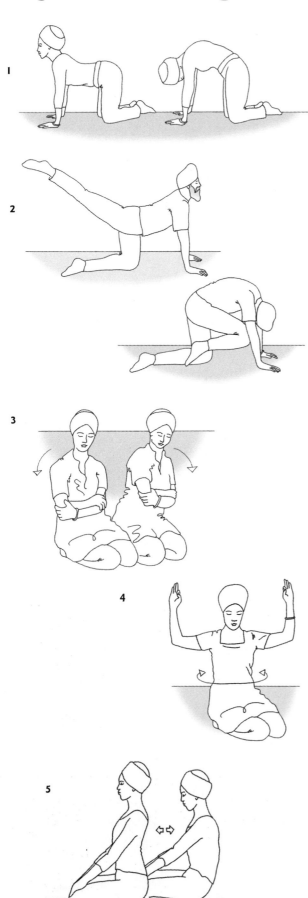

1. **Cat–Cow**: Inhale cow, lift the head and tailbone as you drop the chest. Exhale cat, round the spine as you drop the head and curl the tailbone. Continue for **3 minutes**. Then inhale into Cow Pose and hold 10 seconds. Exhale.

2. **Cow Pose Variation**: In Cow Pose, inhale and raise the right leg and the head up as high as possible. Exhale and swing the knee under the body, and bring the head down. Do **30 repetitions**, then inhale and lift the right leg up, exhale and hold the breath for 10 seconds. Inhale and **repeat with the left leg**. Do 30 repetitions.

3. **Hugging Spinal Bend**: Sit on the heels with knees spread apart. Grasp opposite arms just above the elbows, letting the arms rest against the chest. Bend from side to side in a smooth motion. Inhale center, exhale to each side. 1 minute. Inhale, hold, exhale.

4. **Spinal Twist** variation with **Gyan Mudra**: Still sitting on the heels, raise the arms with the elbows bent at 90° and the upper arms parallel to the floor. Hands in Gyan Mudra, **focus at the Brow Point**, and twist the torso, inhaling left, exhaling right. Powerful breath. **60 swings**. Inhale center, hold the breath, focus. Exhale. Relax.

5. **Spinal Flex**: Bring the knees together and place the hands palm down on the thighs. Focus at the Brow Point, and flex the spine in rhythm with powerful breaths. Do **108 flexes**, then inhale, pull the locks, hold 10 seconds. Exhale and sit still. Meditate silently on the breath—inhaling *Sat*, exhaling *Nam*—for 30 seconds. Inhale, exhale, relax.

6. **Front Bend**: Stand up carefully and shake out the legs. Stand with the feet shoulder-width apart. Hook the thumbs together, palms down. Inhale, raise the arms over the head with the arms hugging the ears. Stretch back, stretching the ribcage and using the full lung capacity. Relax the head back. Exhale forward and bend down, touching the floor, keeping the knees straight. **Repeat 30 times**. Inhale back and hold the stretch a few seconds. Exhale and bend forward at the waist. Let the arms hang down, and completely relax for 30 seconds.

7. **Life Nerve Stretch**: Sit with the legs extended and spread apart. Reach down and grab the toes. Begin stretching, inhale up to the center, exhale down to the left. Inhale up to the center, exhale down to the right. Continue **2 minutes**. Keep the knees straight. Spread the legs further apart and continue for 1 more minute.

8. **Life Nerve Stretch**: Inhale up to the center, hold 3 seconds, then exhale down to the center. Begin stretching down in the center with a continuous pressure and **Long Deep Breathing** for **1 minute**. Inhale and stretch down a bit further. Exhale and come up.

9. **Butterfly**: Bring the soles of the feet together and clasp the fingers around the toes. Keep spine and head straight and begin bouncing the knees up and down. Let the knees move 10″ to 12″. Do vigorously for **1 minute**.

10. **Butterfly Bend**: Hold the same posture, keeping the knees pressed down. Stretch the spine up straight. Inhale up, exhale and bend forward from the waist, bringing the torso down as far as you can. Continue, breathing powerfully for **1 minute**. Inhale up, hold 5 seconds, exhale stretch down and hold for 5 seconds. Relax on the back.

11. **Pelvic Lift**: Still on the back, bend the knees, place the feet flat on the floor near the buttocks, and grab the ankles. Inhale and lift the hips as high as you can, exhale and lower them down. Inhale up, exhale down **24 times**. To end, inhale, stretch up and hold the breath 10 seconds. Relax down and extend the legs straight out.

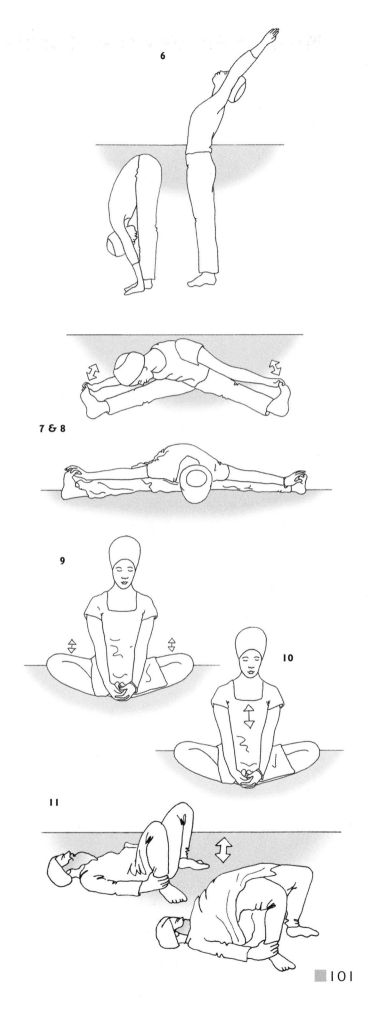

Continued on next page...

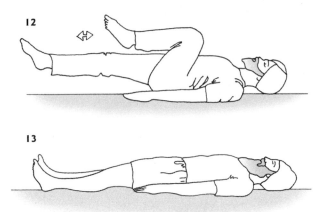

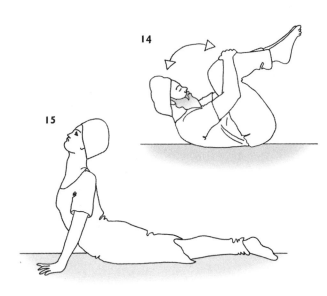

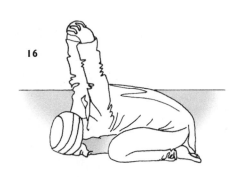

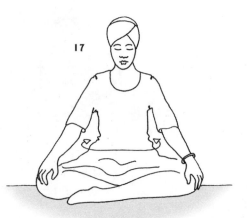

12. **Leg Lifts with Piston Motion**: Lie on the back and point the toes. Lift both legs up together so the heels are 18" above the floor, and begin moving the legs in a piston motion. (This is not a bicycling motion.) Synchronize the motion of the legs with the motion of the breath. One leg moves in as the other moves out. Both legs move simultaneously and the feet move parallel to the floor. Continue for **2 minutes**. Inhale and hold the legs up, extended out for 10 seconds. Exhale and relax on the back.

13. **Corpse Pose**: Relax completely on your back for **1 minute**. Consciously circulate the energy from the Navel Point throughout the body.

14. **Back Rolls**: Bring the knees to the chest, wrap the arms around them, and begin rocking on the spine forward and back. Massage the whole spine for **1-2 minutes**. Then, rock up, turn around and lie down on the stomach.

15. **Cobra Pose**: Stretch up into Cobra Pose. Relax your lower back and buttocks. Focus at the Brow Point, and do **Breath of Fire**. **3 minutes**.
- Inhale, open your eyes, twist left and look at your heels over your left shoulder. Hold 15 seconds. Exhale center.
- Inhale, twist right and look at the heels over the right shoulder. Hold 15 seconds. Exhale.
- Inhale twist left again. Hold 15 seconds. Exhale.
- Inhale, twist right again. Hold 15 seconds. Exhale.
- Inhale center, stretch back and hold 15 seconds. Exhale. Relax down.

16. **Yoga Mudra**: Carefully move into Yoga Mudra. Sitting on your heels, bring your forehead to the floor. Interlace your fingers behind your back and stretch your arms up. Begin **Long Deep Breathing**. Draw the energy into the upper back. **1 minute**. Inhale, hold, exhale. Relax.

17. **Sufi Grind**: Sitting in Easy Pose, hold the kneecaps with the hands. Rotate the middle of the body in circles while keeping the head nearly still. Create a pressure at the base of the spine like a grinding wheel. Use the arms for leverage. **1 minute**. **Reverse direction** and circle for **1 more minute**.

18. **Arm Swings**: Sit in Easy Pose. a) Inhale and draw the elbows back by the sides of the rib cage. Exhale and swing the arms across the chest. b) Inhale again and draw the elbows back by the sides of the rib cage. Exhale and swing the arms up and back over the head. Repeat with a powerful breath and powerful motion for **1-2 minutes**. Inhale, draw the elbows back, stretch the chest forward. Hold 10 seconds. Relax.

19. **Shoulder Shrugs**: Sit with the spine straight and hands on the knees with the elbows relaxed. Inhale and squeeze the shoulders up, exhale and drop them down, using a powerful breath. **108 repetitions**.

20. **Neck Rolls**: Gently circle the head, breathing slowly and deeply, keeping the shoulders relaxed. **1 minute**. Change directions. **1 minute**.

21. **Arm Pumps with Venus Lock**: Sit on the heels and focus at the Brow Point. Join the hands in Venus Lock, with elbows straight. Inhale, bring the arms up 60° above the horizontal. Exhale, bring the arms 60° below the horizontal. Continue inhaling up, exhaling down, powerfully. **70 repetitions**.

22. **Arm Stretch** with Interlaced fingers. Still sitting on the heels, bring the arms up overhead. Flip the hands over so the fingers are interlaced with the palms facing up. Roll the eyes up to the Tenth Gate and focus up above the head. Begin powerful **Breath of Fire for 1 minute**. Then inhale and hold. Focus at the top of the skull at the Tenth Gate. Hold 15 seconds. Relax and carefully bring the arms down.

23. **Meditate**. Come into **Easy Pose**, and sit with a straight spine, one hand on top of the other in your lap, palms up. Meditate silently, inhaling *Sat*, exhaling *Nam*. Sit completely still and consciously expand your aura. Focus deeply. **1 minute**. Inhale, exhale, relax.

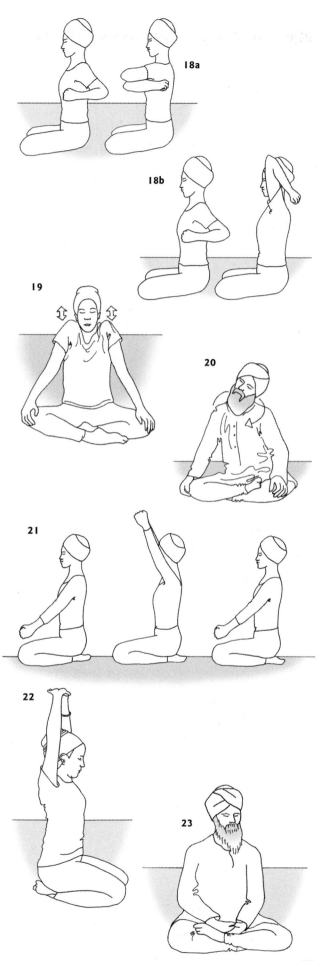

18a

18b

19

20

21

22

23

Beginner's Exercise 1

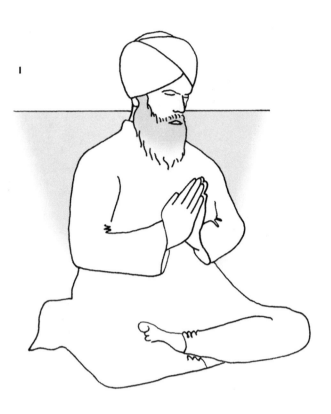

1. Sit in **Easy Pose**. Bring the hands into **Prayer Pose** at the Heart Center. Close the eyelids and concentrate through the Brow Point. Create a positive flow of thought. Project to become healthy, happy, and holy. Continue **7 minutes**.

2. Lie on the back. **Point the toes** forward. Begin **Long Deep Breaths** for **5 minutes**. Then relax for 2 minutes.

3. Still resting on the back, begin **Breath of Fire** for **1 minute**, inhale, hold for 15 seconds and exhale. Take 8 long, deep, complete breaths. **Repeat** this entire sequence **3 times**.

4. Relax for 2 minutes.

5. Lie on the back. Point the toes forward. Lift both legs 6 inches off the ground as you inhale deeply. Hold the position for 15 seconds. Lower the legs. **Repeat five times**.

6. Deeply relax the body, limb-by-limb, organ-by-organ, cell-by-cell for 10 minutes.

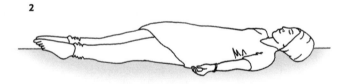

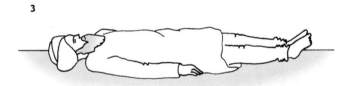

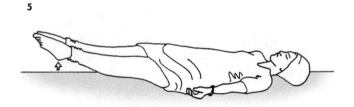

Comments:

This is an easy set to practice for beginners. The effect of the breath is to open the lungs and diaphragm and to slightly stimulate the Navel Center. The stimulation of these two energy resources allows a deep relaxation. This set is excellent for releasing a normal day's tension build-up.

1. Sit on the left heel. Extend the right leg forward, point the toes, and bend forward to grasp them with both hands. Keep the spine as straight as you can and look toward the toes. Hold this position for **2 minutes**, then begin **Breath of Fire for 1 minute**. Switch legs and repeat the exercise. Finish by relaxing for 1 minute.

2. **Bow Pose**: Lie on the stomach, grab the ankles and stretch up. Do **Breath of Fire for 2 minutes**. Relax.

3. **Celibate Pose**: Sit between the heels and raise the arms up to 60° with the palms facing each other. Inhale as you raise the hips up and exhale as you drop down. Bounce up and down consciously and systematically with the breath. **1 minute**. To finish: Exhale deeply and hold the breath out—apply *mulbandh*. Repeat.

4. Stand up. Raise the arms straight up and stretch up on the toes. Bounce up and down on the toes for 5 seconds. Then sit down in Easy Pose. Slowly come back up to standing **without using your hands**. Continue to repeat this cycle for 2 minutes.

5. Sit in Easy Pose with the hands in Gyan Mudra. Go deep within. 5 minutes.

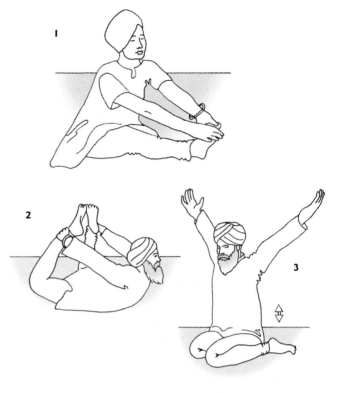

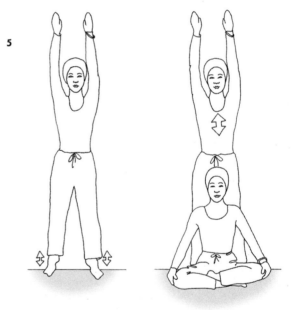

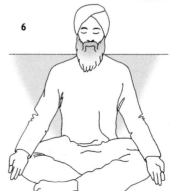

Comments:

This kriya transforms sexual energy into meditative energy. It strengthens the nerves in the upper thighs that regulate sexual potency. Exercises 1 & 2 release the kundalini energy for self-healing; repeat the kriya 2-3 times for a more advanced workout that will make you sweat.

Beginner's Cleansing Set

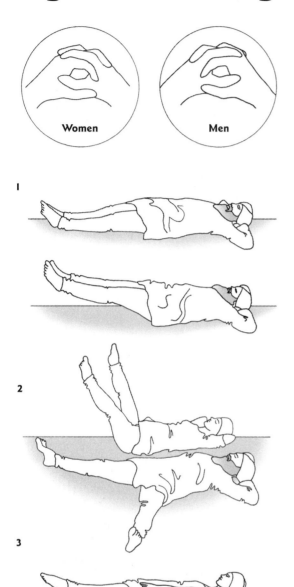

Women   Men

1

2

3

4

1. Lie down on the back and place the hands in **Venus Lock** behind the neck, under any loose hair. Begin **Breath of Fire for 90 seconds**, inhale and hold for 20 seconds. **Repeat Breath of Fire**, inhale and hold for 30 seconds. Relax the breath. To end: Inhale deeply raising both legs one foot from the ground. Hold for 15 seconds, then exhale, inhale, and relax.

2. In this same position, **spread the legs wide**. Begin **Breath of Fire for 1 minute**. Inhale—**raise the legs** 3 feet from the ground and hold for 5 seconds. Relax the legs down. **Repeat 3 times**. To End: Do Breath of Fire for 1 minute, then inhale, raising the legs one foot and hold as long as comfortable. This exercise stimulates the sex energy channels in the upper thigh.

3. **Stretch Pose**: Lie on the back with legs together and raise the heels six inches. Raise the head and shoulders six inches and look at your toes; hands float along the sides of the hips. In this position begin **Breath of Fire** and continue for **3 minutes**. Inhale, exhale and relax.

4. Sit up with the legs extended. Put the left foot on the right thigh. To begin, extend the arms in front of you, hands palm down and parallel to the ground. Inhale, exhale and reach past the toes, extending the hands along the ground. After a good stretch, inhale deeply, sit up and lean back 30°; exhale forward and grab the toes. **Repeat 25 times and switch legs**.

Comments:

This easy series can make you feel light and beautiful. Exercise 1 stimulates the Navel Point energy and circulation of blood in the lungs. Exercise 2 touches the creative power of the sexual energy. Exercise 3 stimulates the Navel Point. Exercise 4 adjusts the chemical balance in the blood and helps

5. Sit up and lean back with the arms behind you for support; the angle of the spine should be about 60° from the ground. Drop the neck back and look at the ceiling, fixing the eyes on one point. Do not wink or blink. Begin **Breath of Fire for 2 minutes**. **Inhale—raise the feet 12 inches** from the ground, keeping the vision steady. Hold for 15–20 seconds, exhale down. **Repeat Breath of Fire for 1 minute**. **Inhale—raise the feet 12 inches**. Hold for 15 seconds. Exhale down and relax completely on the back.

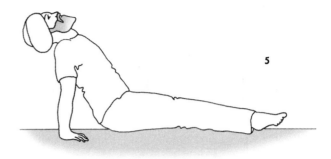

6. Lying on the back, raise your arms to the sky, fingers pointing upward. Inhale deeply and exhale completely bringing your hands into tight fists and slowly moving them down toward the chest. Keep tension in the arms as if struggling to pull a 1,000-pound weight; if you apply sufficient tension, the fists will shake as they touch the chest. Inhale deep and repeat the exercise with the breath held in.

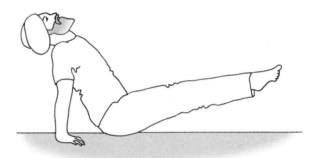

7. Deeply and completely relax for 5 minutes.

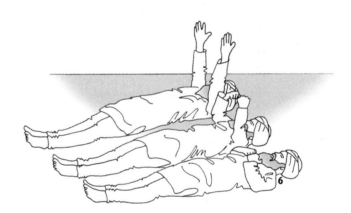

the lower back and waistline. Exercise 5 moves the energy into the brain and eyes. It has helped cases of headaches and eye diseases such as cataract. Exercise 6 removes any residual tension and allows you to relax.

Kriya for Lungs, Magnetic Field and Deep Meditation

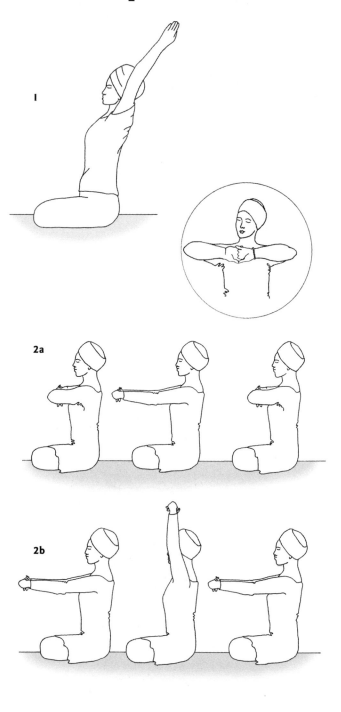

1. Sit in **Easy Pose**. Stretch the arms overhead with the palms together in **Prayer Pose**. Arch the spine as far up and back as possible. Begin **Long Deep Breathing** through the **mouth—whistle** on both the inhale and the exhale. **5 Minutes**. Relax.

2. Stretch the arms straight out in front of you with the fingers interlaced, palms facing outward. a) Inhale in this position, exhale and bring the hands toward the chest. Continue in a fairly rapid motion, about one per second, for 2 minutes. b) Then, inhale and stretch the arms out in front of you, suspend the breath as you extend the arms overhead and back down to parallel (this is fairly rapid); exhale bring the hands toward the chest. Continue this sequence for **2 minutes**. Then go immediately to the next exercise.

3. Without resting, stretch the arms in the shape of a V in front of you (about a 60° angle to each other). Inhale, suspend the breath and make fists with the hands. **With a great deal of tension**, bring the fists to the chest. Exhale—release the hands and arms back to the 60° angle. Your face should be angry throughout the exercise. **3 minutes**.

Comments:

This series begins by purifying the blood and expanding the lung capacity. Then the circulatory system is stimulated. The Throat Chakra and the correlated functioning of the thyroid and parathyroid

4. Place the hands behind the neck with the fingers interlaced and the palms facing up. Inhale—stretch the arms up straight. Exhale—relax them down behind the neck. **2 minutes**.

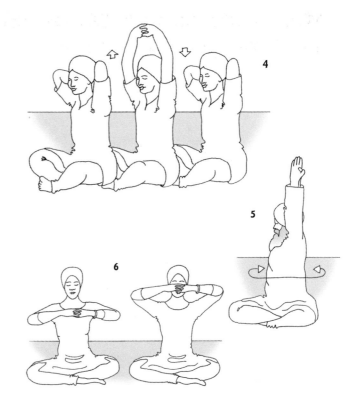

5. Stretch the arms up straight overhead with the palms together, thumbs locked (or crossed). **Inhale** and twist to the **left**; **exhale** and twist to the **right**. Fairly rapid pace. **2 minutes**.

6. Interlace the fingers with the palms down in front of the chest. Inhale—bring the hands up to the eye level; exhale—bring the hands back to the chest. Fairly rapid pace. **2 minutes**.

7. **Spinal Twist**: Bring the hands to the shoulders, fingers in front, thumbs in back. Inhale—twist to the left; exhale—twist to the right. **2 minutes**.

8. **Shoulder Shrugs**: Sit in Easy Pose. Place the hands on the knees. Inhale and shrug the shoulders up. Exhale down. **2 minutes**. Without a break, **move immediately into Spine Flex**.

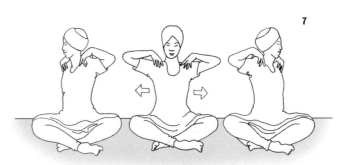

9. **Spine Flex**: Still in Easy Pose, flex the spine forward and back. Inhale—press the chest forward; exhale—extend it back. **2 minutes**. Roll the eyes up as far as possible. Concentrate at the crown of the head.

10. Meditate. 15 minutes.

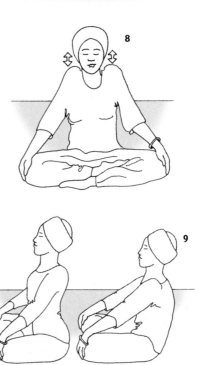

secretions are optimized. The circulation is increased and the upper magnetic field of the body is enlarged. This is an excellent preparation for beginners who want to learn deep meditation.

Surya Kriya

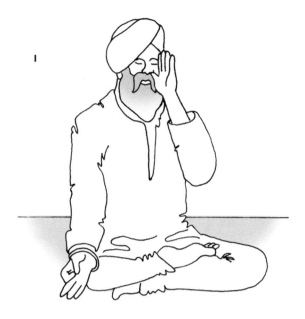

1. **Right Nostril Breathing**: Sit in Easy Pose with a straight spine. Rest the right hand in Gyan Mudra on the knee. Block the left nostril with the thumb of the left hand. The other four fingers point straight up. Begin long, deep, powerful breaths in and out of the right nostril. Focus on the flow of the breath. Continue for **3–5 minutes**. Inhale, exhale and relax.

2. **Sat Kriya**: Sit on the heels. Raise the arms over the head, elbows straight, palms together. Interlace the fingers except for the index fingers, which point straight up. Men cross the right thumb over the left with the left little finger on the bottom; women cross left thumb over right, right pinkie on bottom. Chant *Sat* as you pull the navel in and *Nam* as you release the navel. Focus at the Brow Point. Continue for **3 minutes**. Then inhale—hold the breath. Apply *mulbandh* and imagine your energy radiating from the Navel Point and circulating throughout the body. Relax. **Repeat Sat Kriya for 3 minutes**. Then inhale, apply *mulbandh*, and mentally draw all the energy to the top of the fingertips. Exhale and relax.

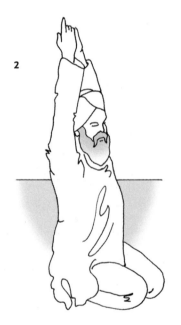

3. **Spine Flex with *mulbandh***: Sit in Easy Pose. Grasp the shins with both hands. Inhale—flex the spine forward and lift the chest. Exhale—extend the spine backwards. Keep the Neck Lock and the head level throughout. On each inhale mentally vibrate the mantra *Sat*, on the exhale vibrate *Nam*. On each exhale apply *mulbandh*. Continue rhythmically with deep breaths **108 times**. Then inhale—hold briefly with the spine perfectly straight. Exhale and relax.

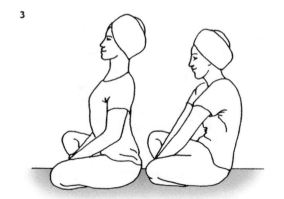

Comments:

This kriya is named after the energy of the sun. When you have a lot of "sun energy" you do not get cold, you are energetic, expressive, extroverted and enthusiastic. It is the energy of purification. It helps you maintain a healthy weight, aids digestion, and makes the mind clear, analytical, and action-oriented. The exercises systematically stimulate the positive *pranic* force and the kundalini energy itself. Exercise 1 draws on the "sun breath" and gives you a clear, focused mind. Exercise 2 is for the release of the energy stored at the Navel Point. Exercise 3 brings the

4. **Frog Pose**: Squat down so the buttocks are on the heels. The heels are off the ground and touching each other. Put the fingertips on the ground between the knees with the head up. Inhale, raise the buttocks high and let the head drop, keeping the fingers on the ground. Exhale, come down, lift the head and let the buttocks strike the heels. The exhale should be strong. Continue with deep breaths **26 times**. Inhale up, then relax down, sitting on the heels.

5. In **Rock Pose**, place the hands on the thighs. With the spine very straight, inhale deeply and turn the head to the left. Mentally vibrate *Sat*. Exhale completely as you turn the head to the right. Mentally vibrate *Nam*. Continue inhaling and exhaling for **3 minutes**. Then inhale with the head straight forward. Exhale and relax.

6. **Sit in Easy Pose**. Put the hands on the shoulders with the fingers in front and the thumbs in the back. The upper arms and elbows are parallel to the ground. Inhale as you bend to the left, exhale and bend to the right. Continue this swaying motion with deep breaths for **3 minutes**. Then inhale center. Exhale and relax.

7. Sit in a perfect meditative posture with the spine straight. Direct all your attention through the Brow Point. Pull the Navel Point in—hold it—apply *mulbandh*. Watch the flow of breath. On the inhale listen to the silent *Sat* on the exhale listen to the silent *Nam*. Continue **6 minutes** or more.

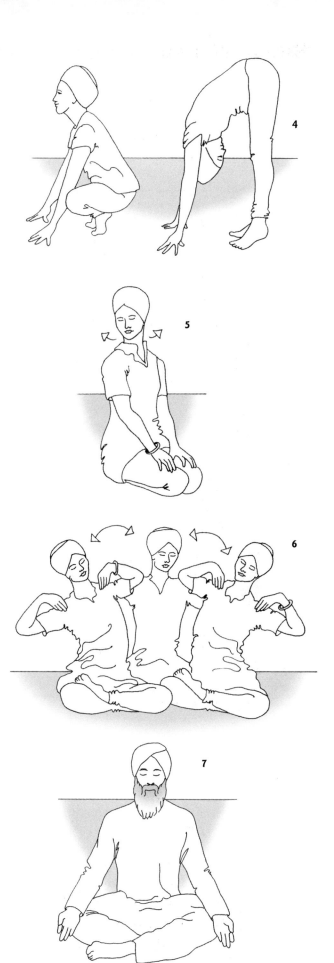

released kundalini energy along the path of the spine and aids its flexibility. Exercise 4 transforms the sexual energy. Exercise 5 opens the Throat Chakra, stimulates circulation to the head and works on the thyroid and parathyroid glands. Exercise 6 flexes the spine, distributes the energy over the whole body, and balances the magnetic field. Exercise 7 takes you into a deep self-healing meditation. This Kriya should occasionally be included in your regular sadhana practice to build strength and the ability to focus on multiple tasks.

Apana Kriya (Elimination Exercises)

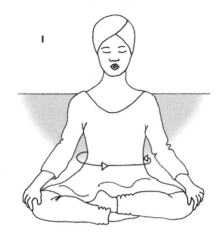

1. **Vatskar Kriya:** Sit in Easy Pose with hands on the knees. Make a beak of the mouth and drink as much air as you can into the stomach using short, continuous sips, as if you were swallowing. Pull in and hold. Roll the stomach to the left, when the breath has been held in for half its maximum time, reverse the direction to the right. Continue rolling the stomach as long as possible with Neck Lock applied. When the breath can be held in no longer, straighten the spine and exhale slowly (not powerfully) through the nose. Repeat the complete exercise 2 times. Note: Always do this on an empty stomach and not more than twice per day.

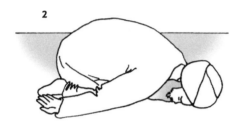

2. **Baby Pose:** Sit on the heels and touch the forehead to the ground. Place the hands palm up by the hips. Imagine that there is a big, 100-pound tail coming off the end of the spine and wag it as if trying to make it break the wall. Move the hips left and right—a few inches—as if the tailbone traces out a "U"; this will churn the navel and the lower abdomen as you move. Continue for **3 minutes** followed by 5 minutes of rest.

3. Lie down on the back. Press the toes forward. Lift the legs three feet. Start **Long Deep Breathing**. Continue for **2 or 3 minutes**. Inhale—hold briefly and relax.

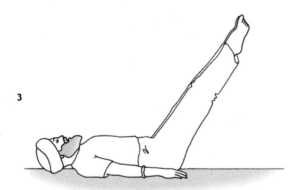

4. Lie down on the back, bring the legs overhead and catch the toes. Roll back and forth from the base of the spine to the neck. Hold onto the toes and keep rocking for **3 minutes**.

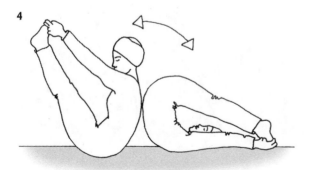

Comments:

This is a good example of a simple but powerful series that was kept secret by those few yogis who learned it. This will allow you to completely master your digestive system and give a youthful appearance to your skin. Aging does not start just with years; it begins with nutritional deficiency, intestinal problems, untended emotional and physical stress and an inflexible spine that disrupts the flow of meridians as well as the rejuvenating flow of your spinal fluid.

5. **Alternate Nostril Breath**: Sit up immediately in **Easy Pose**. As calmly as possible, bring the right thumb to the right nostril to close it off. Inhale through the left nostril, using the little finger, close off the left nostril and exhale through the right. Continue for **3 minutes**, then inhale and feel the energy radiate throughout the body, giving health and life.

6. Sit in Easy Pose. Place the **Venus Lock** a few inches in front of the chest at the **Heart Center** with the palms facing the chest. Inhale and turn the head to the left; exhale and turn the head to the right. Continue for **3 minutes**.

7. Sit in Easy Pose. Stretch the arms out to the sides, parallel to the ground. Swing the arms back in a rolling motion as if swimming. Continue for **1 minute**.

8. To end: Inhale and hold the breath as you bend the elbows, bringing the fingertips onto the shoulders. This magnetizes the electric current. While the breath is held, the energy starts circulating. Exhale— let the energy flow to all parts of the body and feel refreshed.

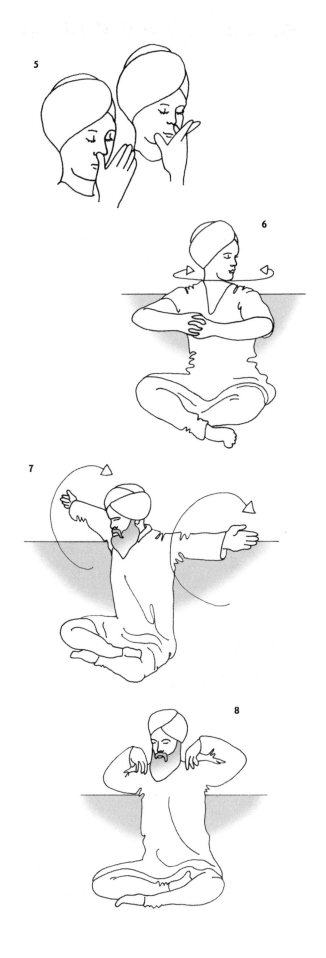

Exercise 1 adjusts the acid–alkaline balance in the stomach, but it must be done regularly without missing a single day. Exercise 2 strengthens the heart; Exercise 3 slims the waistline and cleans the gallbladder; Exercise 4 flushes the circulation and balances the nerves. Exercises 5 and 6 distribute the *pranic* force and stimulate the thyroid and parathyroid. Exercise 7 strengthens the psycho-magnetic field of the aura.

Life Nerve Stimulation

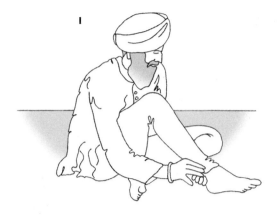

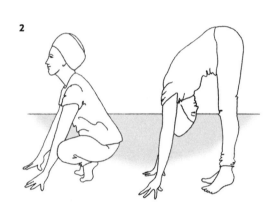

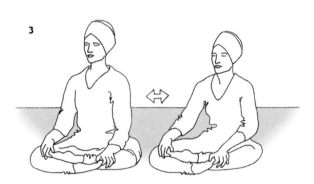

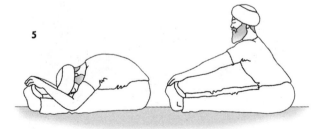

1. Sit in a comfortable pose and massage the Achilles tendon with the thumbs of both hands. The area to rub is from the heel up the tendon about 4 inches. If you press correctly, the toes will flex slightly. Rub the tendon of each foot firmly and rhythmically for **2 minutes on each side**.

2. **Frog Pose**: Squat down so the buttocks are on your heels. The heels are off the ground and touching each other. Put the fingertips on the ground between the knees. Keep the head up. Inhale, raise the buttocks high and let the head drop, keeping the fingers on the ground. Exhale, come down, lift the head and let the buttocks strike the heels. The exhale should be strong. Continue this cycle for **3–5 minutes**.

3. Sit in a comfortable cross-legged pose. **Grasp the big toe** of each foot with your hands. Using the thumb tip or knuckle of the thumb, press the fleshy part of the big toes with 10–15 lbs. of pressure. Keep the pressure strong and constant. Begin to **flex the spine**. Inhale—flex the spine forward. Exhale and extend the spine backwards. Continue rhythmically with deep breaths for **3 minutes**. Then inhale, hold briefly, and relax the breath.

4. **Repeat Frog Pose**: 3–5 minutes.

5. Stretch both legs out straight in front on the ground. Bend forward and grasp the toes with both hands. Pull back on the toes for 30 seconds. Then hold onto the toes as you inhale—arch up, then exhale—bend forward. **Pump the spine** up-and-down with the breath. Do **26** of these **pumps** with deep breaths. To end: Inhale—extend the spine up and arch the head back. Exhale and relax the breath.

Comments:

This kriya invigorates the heart and gives energy to the regenerative and sexual system. Rubbing near the heels breaks up long-term crystal (calcium deposit) build-up. This in turn helps improve circulation to the legs. Two complete cycles of this kriya at maximum times is a good workout.

1. **Triangle Pose** (Down Dog) with leg extended. Start on your hands and knees. From this position, lift the hips so that the body forms a triangle. Raise the right leg up with the knee straight so your spine and extended leg form a line. Exhale—bend the elbows and bring the head forward and down toward the ground. Inhale—lift up. Continue this triangle push-up for **90 seconds**. **Switch legs** and continue for another **90 seconds**.

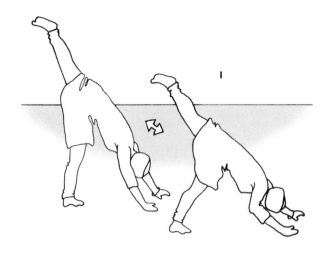

2. Sit in Easy Pose. Extend the left arm forward, parallel to the ground with the palm facing to the right. Bring the right arm, with the palm facing down, beneath the left wrist. From this position, drop the thumb side of the hand down and turn the right hand so that the palm faces the back of the left hand. With both palms facing the right, lock the fingers of the right hand down over the left and the fingers of the left hand down over the right. Inhale—raise the arms to 60°. Exhale—bring the arms down to the starting point, extended parallel to the ground. Keep the elbows straight. Breathe deeply for **2 to 3 minutes**. Then inhale—stretch the arms up and relax.

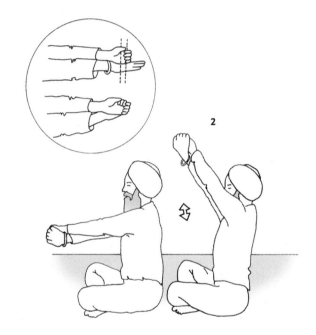

3. Sit in Easy Pose. Extend the arms forward, parallel to the ground with the palms facing each other about 6 inches apart. As you inhale, let the arms drop back and stretch toward each other. Exhale—bring them forward to the original position. This feels like a natural swing as the arms go back and down then snap back forward. The shoulders stay relaxed through the swing at about 8 swings per 10 seconds. Continue **3 minutes** with a deep rhythmic breath.

Comments:

This is a great kriya for keeping disease away and developing your aura. The time can be built up to 7 ½ minutes for each side in Exercise 1; and 15 minutes each for Exercises 2 and 3. This will create a tremendous sweat. It will rid you of almost any digestive problem. It gives strength to the arms and it extends the power of protection and projection in the personality.

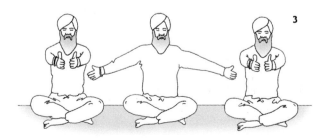

Strength to Sacrifice

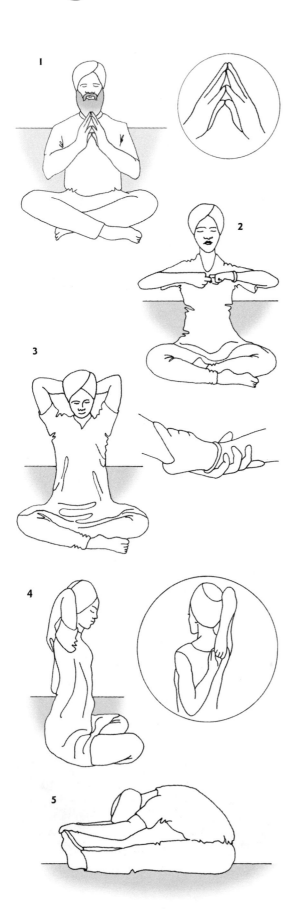

1. Sit in **Easy Pose** with the spine straight and the chest lifted. Put the fingertips together, pointing up, to form a tent. Hold this mudra at the level of the chin. Chant "God and me, me and God are One." Keep the fingers pressed tightly together as you chant. Continue for **3–6 minutes**.

2. Lock the middle fingers of both hands together at chest level. Pull the fingers as hard as you can. Be constant. Hold for **90 seconds**.

3. In Easy Pose with a straight spine, grasp both wrists with the opposite hands. Place this lock behind the neck and pull the hands and forearms down. Hold the position with Long Deep Breathing for **3 minutes**.

4. Drop the right hand behind the upper spine and bring the left hand behind you at the level of the Heart Center, with the palm facing away; grasp the fingertips of each hand. Then inhale, exhale deeply, hold the breath out and pull the Navel Lock tightly. Repeat the breath and lock cycle for **3 minutes**.

5. **Forward Bend**: Extend the legs. Bend forward and grab the toes. Hold as still as a rock for 10 seconds. Then relax.

Comments:

The capacity to transcend is required of the yogi and the saint. For this the nerves must be strong and balanced. The circumvent magnetic force of the aura must be so strong that no negativity can enter your field and provoke a reaction. Instead this kriya helps you stay strong based in your consciousness. There are many challenges and lessons in life. One teacher is like Jupiter—jovial, expansive and inspirational. The other teacher is like Saturn—heavy, direct and painful. No one likes the Saturnine lessons of life, and yet painful situations are often the best teacher and the ones that force the greatest transformation and re-evaluation within us. Our natural tendency is to escape to avoid being trapped by commitment, or to lessen our pains by only hearing what we want to hear. This kriya gives you the calm, assertive stillness to tolerate the minor pains, learn from the great ones and make Saturn your friend. Yogi Bhajan gave us seven steps to happiness. The last step is the power to sacrifice. That capacity allows us to transcend, to be part of something greater and to balance our short-term needs with our long-term destiny.

1. Sit in **Easy Pose** with a straight spine. Place the hands on the knees in **Gyan Mudra**. Keep the elbows straight. Close the eyes and focus deeply. Inhale and exhale deeply. This cycle will take about 8 seconds. Take a total of 12 breaths. On the thirteenth breath cycle, exhale completely and hold the breath out. Pump the stomach in and out at a moderate pace. (You may add a mentally repeated *Sat* as you pull the belly in, and *Nam* as you relax it.) When you can no longer hold the breath out, inhale and repeat the exercise. Continue for **3 minutes**.

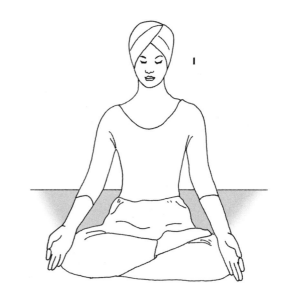

2. Stretch the legs forward. Keeping the spine erect, bring the right foot to the groin, on top of the left thigh at the level of the hip. Bend forward at the waist and grasp the toes of the left foot with both hands. Keep the spine as straight as you can and look toward the toes. Breathe deeply; **constrict the tip of your nose** as if you were "sniffing." Continue for **3 minutes**. Then inhale, hold briefly, exhale and relax.

3. Sit straight and meditate on the calm flow of the breath. Briefly visualize your spine from the base to the top and then to the Brow Point. Relax and meditate.

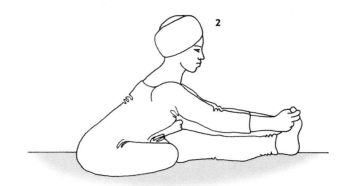

Comments:

This kriya helps you gain endurance and constancy. The first exercise stimulates the navel center and digestion. The second exercise gives energy to the upper body and stretches the life nerves in the legs. The third allows the energy changes to stabilize and consolidate themselves.

In life, we must increase our wisdom and experience so we can live as householders but with higher consciousness. The yogi's aim is to live with maximum light and effectiveness but also be very humble. This is why a teacher remains a student throughout his life and grows more humble with age. This kriya lets the Self take care of the gross self so that the physical body can have the energy to carry out the Self's desires. Regular practice of this kriya helps balance the difference between your inner reality and your expression. A good way to practice this kriya is to repeat the set 3 or 4 times, then deeply relax for 5–10 minutes.

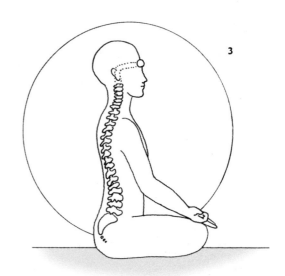

Kriya for Tolerance

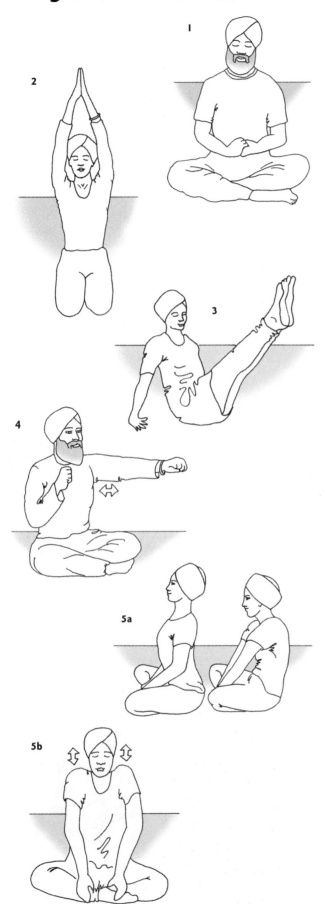

1. Sit in Easy Pose with the spine straight. Lock the fingertips into **Bear Grip** with the **right palm facing down**. Push the side of the hands into the Navel Point as you exhale completely. Hold the breath out, then inhale and hold the breath for 7 to 8 seconds. Continue this cycle for **3 minutes**.

2. **Sat Kriya with palms flat**: Sit on the heels and raise the arms overhead with palms flat together. Men cross the right thumb over the left; women cross left thumb over right. Pull in the Navel Point as you say *Sat*, relax the Navel Point as you say *Nam*. Continue for **3 minutes**.

3. Stretch the legs out straight in front of you. Place the palms on the ground behind you. Raise both legs to 60° and hold this position with **Breath of Fire**. Continue for **2 minutes**. To end: Inhale, exhale, apply *mulbandh* Then relax immediately into Easy Pose and **belly laugh loudly for 1 minute**.

4. In Easy Pose, bring your hands into fists at the shoulders. Inhale deeply and suspend the breath, begin punching forward (as in boxing) with alternate hands. When you must, exhale, and inhale deeply to continue. **3 minutes**.

5. Sit in Easy Pose. **Alternate between Camel Ride and Shoulder Shrugs**: a) put the hands on the shins and inhale—flex the spine forward; exhale—extend it back. b) Inhale—lift the shoulders up to the ears; exhale—drop the shoulders down. The pace is about 5 full cycles in 10 seconds. Continue this cycle with deep breaths for **3 minutes**. Then inhale, exhale completely, apply *mulbandh*. Relax.

Comments:

To gain strength for tolerance and humility, the navel center needs to be developed. This kriya works on the abdomen, stimulating the navel energy to rise to the higher centers and then integrating it with the whole aura. It is a good preparation for meditation. Two cycles of this kriya give you a good physical tune-up.

Breath Meditation Series for Glandular Balance

1. Sit in Easy Pose. Break your inhale and exhale into **16 segments**—short sniffs. With each segment of the breath, both inhale and exhale, mentally vibrate Sat Nam, and pull the Navel Point slightly. Start with **5 minutes**. Then add 1 minute each day to a maximum of 31 minutes per day.

2. Lie on your back. Put the arms straight overhead on the ground with the palms up. Inhale—raise both legs 6 inches. Exhale—let the legs release down and bring the chin to the chest. Continue with Long Deep Breathing for **3 minutes**. Rest for 2 minutes.

3. Sit in Easy Pose. Grab opposite elbows, with your arms across the chest. Inhale—in the upright position. Exhale—bend forward and place the forehead on the ground. Continue for **3 minutes** with Long Deep Breathing.

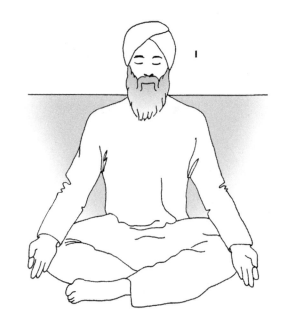

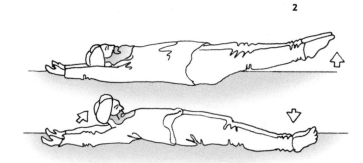

Comments:

Your glands are the guardians of your physical health and your stability in infinite consciousness. Their secretions determine the chemistry of the blood and the blood, in turn, determines the composition of your personality. If, for example, you lack proper iodine in the thyroid gland or have too much thyroxin produced, you will lack patience and seldom succeed in staying calm and cool.

If you are to gain mastery of unlimited consciousness in yourself, you must master the physical consciousness to help you, not hinder you. It is best to work on this while you are young. Once you are old, it is much more difficult because the bodies responsiveness decreases naturally. Prepare your glandular balance in your youth so that age, disease, and fatigue don't blunt your experience of God-consciousness.

If you keep the first exercise to 5 minutes, then repeat the kriya 3 times in order to have a thorough glandular workout.

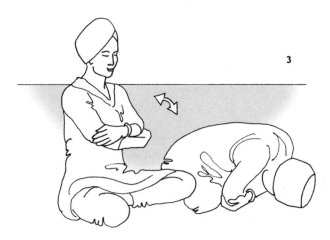

Purifying the Self

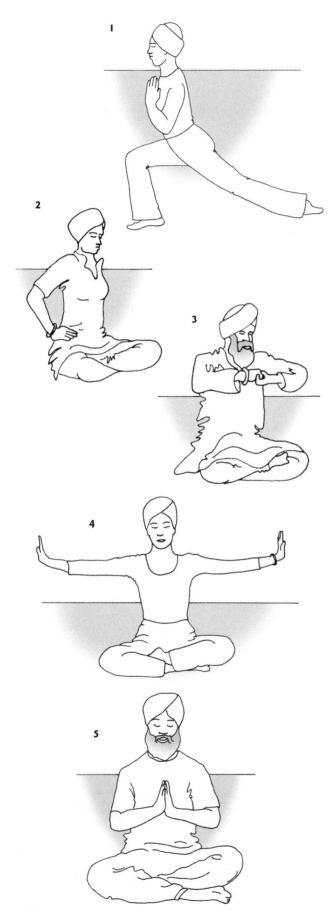

1. Stand up. Extend one leg back as far as you can with the top of the foot on the ground; the opposite knee bends until the thigh is almost parallel with the ground. Most of the pressure will be on the bent leg. Put the palms together at the center of the chest. Focus at the Brow Point.

In this position, **take three deep breaths**, holding the inhalation for about 8 seconds each time. Come back to standing and **switch to the opposite leg and take three deep breaths** on this side, holding the inhalation for about 8 seconds each time. Repeat twice more on each side.

2. Sit in Easy Pose. Place the hands on the hips. Lift the diaphragm high. Raise both shoulders as high as possible. Inhale and exhale very deeply while holding this posture. Continue **2–3 minutes**.

3. Sit in Easy Pose, and bring the hands into **Bear Grip** (hook the fingers together at the center of the chest) with the right palm facing down. Forearms and elbows are parallel to the ground. Inhale deeply. Exhale forcefully and completely and apply *mulbandh*. Inhale—hold the breath, apply *mulbandh* and mentally raise the *pranic* energy from the base of the spine to the crown. Continue this breath cycle for **3 minutes**.

4. Sit in Easy Pose. Extend the arms out the sides, parallel to the ground. Press the palms out with the fingers pointing up. Roll the eyes up and focus at the Brow Point. Inhale deeply—hold the breath while applying a firm *mulbandh* for 20 seconds. Then exhale and repeat. Continue for **2–3 minutes**.

5. In Easy Pose, press the palms together—about 2–3 inches in front of the chest—with the fingers pointing up. Pull the spine straight. Press with 30–50 pounds of pressure. Hold the position for **2 minutes**. Then relax.

Comments:

This kriya energizes you and helps purify the mind and body. It is an excellent kriya to prepare yourself before giving a healing, relaxing massage to someone. If you are a professional massage therapist, it can help you sustain your energy and prevent you from getting drained. The exercise sequence guides energy up along the spine, opens the chakras and then expands the aura. Exercise 1 will raise the sexual and digestive energies of the body. Exercise 2 takes energy past the Diaphragm Lock and opens the lungs and Throat Center. Exercise 3 opens the heart and the central channel of the spine. Exercises 4 and 5 increase healing power in the hands, circulation to the upper body, and steadiness of concentration.

Disease Resistance and Heart Helper

1. Sit in Easy Pose. Interlace the fingers of both hands. Press the thumb tips together. Place this mudra with palms up in the lap. Apply *mulbandh* and chant "God and me, me and God are one." With each cycle of the mantra, pull up the locks a little tighter. Continue for **3 minutes**.

2. Sit in Easy Pose with the hands in Gyan Mudra resting on the knees. Inhale deeply, exhale slowly and completely **without dropping the rib cage.** Hold the breath out and pump the stomach. When you cannot pump anymore, inhale, exhale and continue the same pattern for **3 minutes**.

3. Sit in Easy Pose. Bring the left hand behind the back, stretching it toward the right shoulder. The palm faces away from the body. The right hand is in Gyan Mudra at the knee. Inhale deeply, exhale completely. Apply *mulbandh*. Hold the breath out as long as you can. Then inhale and repeat the cycle. Continue **3–5 minutes**.

4. Sit in any comfortable meditation posture. Meditate on the regular energetic flow of the breath. Feel your radiance and light.

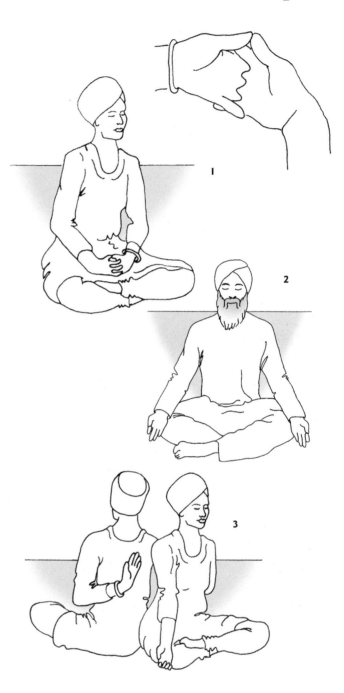

Comments:

The first exercise improves your health by invigorating the First Chakra and elimination. It promotes calmness and disease resistance. The second exercise stimulates the Third Chakra, increases endurance and nerve strength. The third exercise strengthens the heart and increases circulation above the diaphragm. Three repetitions of this kriya is a very effective practice.

Circulatory Systems and Magnetic Field

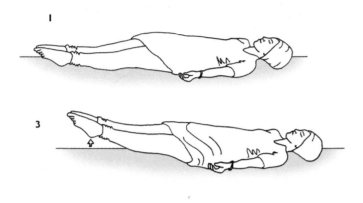

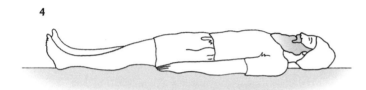

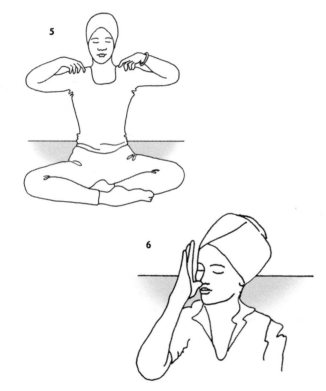

1. Lie on the back, arms straight along the side of the body, heels and toes together. **Press the toes forward**. Continue pressing the toes deeper and deeper for 1 minute, then **lift the heels six inches**. Begin Long Deep Breathing. Keep the head relaxed down on the ground and continue for **3 minutes**.

2. Dead relaxation for **2 minutes**.

3. Repeat Exercise 1. Press the toes as hard as you possibly can. Hold for 1 minute, then lift the heels up **three inches only**. Apply *mulbandh*. Relax.

4. Dead relaxation. Become disassociated from the body. Imagine that you have no legs, no arms, no trunk, no head. Continue for **2 minutes**.

5. Sit in Easy Pose. Put hands your hands on your shoulders; fingers in front, thumbs in back. Begin **Long Deep Breathing for 3 minutes**. To end: Inhale and mentally circulate the *pranic* energy. Exhale and relax.

6. **Left Nostril Breathing**: Make an antenna of the right hand with the fingers pointing straight up in the air and the thumb closing off the right nostril. Begin Long Deep Breathing through the left nostril for **5 minutes**. Inhale—hold for 30 seconds and let the energy circulate in the body. Exhale.

Comments:

Blood is the lifeline to your cells. Do you know that the blood cells act differently with different magnetic influences? Exercises 1–4 raise and lower the blood pressure and increase circulation to the limbs and head. Exercises 5–7 magnetize and charge the

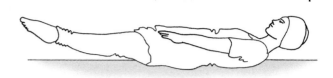

7. **Stretch Pose**: Lie on the back. Lift toes and head 12 inches from the ground. **Keep Up!** Breathe naturally for 2 minutes; then begin Breath of Fire for 1 more minute to relieve pain. Inhale—hold, and relax.

8. Deep relaxation to a gong or to the chanting of Long Sat Nam (see Basic Breath Series), or any beautiful divine version of the Ashtang Mantra can be done. Relax for **10 minutes**. Then rotate the wrists and ankles and stretch the spine.

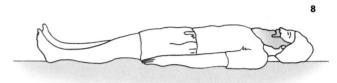

9. **Bundle Roll**. Lie with hands at sides and legs straight and stiff. Begin rolling. Imagine the body is a bundle of logs tied together; roll over and over—without using the arms or legs.

10. Without a rest, lie flat on the back, **open the mouth, and laugh loudly**. Release the energy through the lungs. Relax for 1 minute and then **laugh again**. Relax.

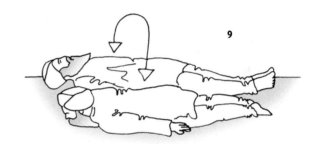

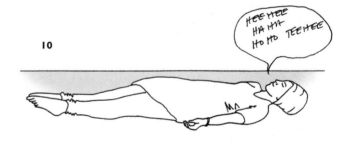

blood with pranic force. This is like getting a transfusion of fresh young blood. The last exercise allows the new energy to circulate and affect the entire body. With the bundle roll, you consolidate those effects as you strengthen the navel for the rest of the day.

Magnetic Field and Heart Center

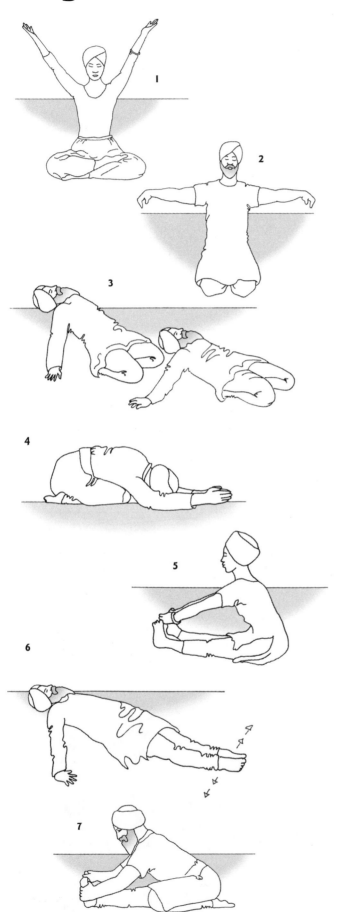

1. Sit in Easy Pose. Raise the arms to a 60° angle with wrists and elbows straight, palms facing up. Begin **Breath of Fire for 1 minute**. Then inhale—suspend the breath and pump the stomach **16 times**. Exhale—relax the breath. Continue this cycle of pumping the navel on the inhale then exhaling for **2 or 3 minutes**.

2. Immediately sit on the heels with arms stretched out to the sides, parallel to the ground. Let the hands hang limp from the wrists. Begin **Breath of Fire for 3 minutes**. Inhale—suspend, exhale and relax.

3. Sit on the heels. Spread the knees wide and lean back 60° from the ground. Support the body with your arms behind you. Tilt the head back—**inhale**—**pump the navel** in and out until the breath can be held no longer. Exhale. Continue for **1½ to 2 minutes**. Then, tilt the spine back further to 30° and continue the breathing cycle for another **1½ to 2 minutes**.

4. Still sitting on the heels with knees spread, put the forehead on the ground with arms stretched forward and relaxed in Gurpranam. Keep this posture and, after 1 minute, begin Long Deep Breathing for 2 minutes. Then for 2 minutes **chant in call and response style**:

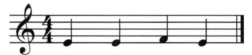

Teacher: **Ong, ong, ong, ong.**
Class: **Ong, ong, ong, ong**
Teacher: **Sohung, sohung. sohung, sohung**
Class: **Sohung, sohung, sohung, sohung**

5. Rise up, stretch the legs out straight in front and spread them slightly. Come into **Forward Bend**, reaching for the toes. Hold for **1 minute**.

6. **Back Platform**: Sit up straight, legs still extended. Place the hands slightly behind the hips, fingertips pointing towards the toes, and lift the hips off the ground. The body forms a straight line from the toes to the chest. Keep the arms straight and drop the head back. Begin **Breath of Fire**. After 30 seconds, begin to walk the legs apart until they are spread wide, then walk them back together again, continuing Breath of Fire for 30 more seconds. To end: Inhale, exhale and move immediately into a Front Stretch holding the toes for 1 minute. Relax on the back for 3 minutes.

7. Sit on the left heel, stretch the right leg forward and grab the big toe with the right hand. Pulling back on the toe, grab the heel with the left hand. Keep a strong Neck Lock (*jalandhar bandh*) and the eyes fixed on the big toe. Inhale deeply—exhale and pull the Root Lock (*mulbandh*) and the Diaphragm Lock (*uddiyana bandh*)—hold the breath out for 8 seconds keeping

the locks pulled tightly. This is **Maha Mudra**. Release the locks and inhale. Continue for **3 minutes**. Then **relax for 5 minutes** on the back.

8. Still on the back, stretch the arms overhead on the ground. Raise the left leg 90° and begin **Breath of Fire for 1 minute**. Continue Breath of Fire and switch sides, raising the right leg 90° for **1 minute**. Continue Breath of Fire and lift both legs to 12 inches for **1 minute**. Relax for 2 minutes.

9. Slowly come into **Shoulder Stand**. Spread the legs wide and begin **Breath of Fire for 3 minutes. Relax** on the back for **3 minutes**.

10. Lie on the back. Bring the arms up to 90°, palms facing each other and fingertips pointing up. Inhale and lift both legs 6 inches. On the exhale, lower the legs and bring the head up, pressing the chin to the chest. Continue **3 minutes** with Long Deep Breathing. **Relax 2 minutes**.

11. Sit in Easy Pose and hold opposite elbows across the chest. Roll the head in a slow figure eight for 30 seconds in one direction, then 30 seconds in the other direction.

Then inhale deeply, and bend forward to the ground. Continue inhaling as you bow and exhaling as you rise up; move as fast as possible. **10 times**.

12. Meditate by chanting:

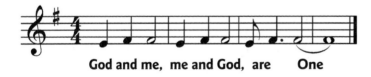

God and me, me and God, are One

Comments:

    This set works on coordination and repair of the nervous system by stimulating the Heart Center. Your normal feeling of happiness, connection, and well-being depend on the balance of your individual psycho-electromagnetic field. If it is strong, your muscles can accurately respond to and use the sensory input from all the nerves; your perceptual acuity will be at its best. Proper maintenance of the nerves depends on the basic elements and hormones in the constitution of the blood. This set will balance the blood.

    Exercise 1 builds the psycho-electromagnetic field. If your elbows bend, the psycho-electromagnetic field will not be reformed and strengthened properly. If the exhale after pumping the stomach is rough or gasping,

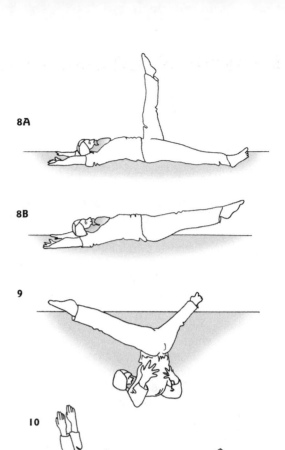

8A

8B

9

10

11

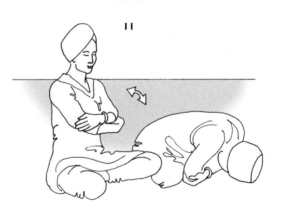

Continued on next page...

Magnetic Field and Heart Center

then your magnetic field is very weak. Exercise 2 is for the heart. This stimulates the thyroid, parathyroid and Navel Center. If you practice these, you will never need cosmetics. A smooth, radiant complexion and a glow in the eyes and face is a natural by-product of this exercise.

Exercise 4 stimulates the circulation of blood into the brain and moves the spinal fluid. This helps repair the damage to the brain done by drugs like alcohol, marijuana, etc. Exercise 5 is for balance; exercise 6 is for the thyroid, lower back and heart. Exercise 7 is Maha Mudra—the great seal of yoga. Its effects fill pages in the ancient texts on yoga. This exercise can be practiced by itself. Exercise 8 balances prana and apana. Exercise 9 is for the thyroid and 10 and 11 are for the Heart Center.

The best results are always obtained if you practice a set until you master it. If you cannot do the exercises for the full time period, do what you can and slowly build up to it. When you can keep up on all the given times and are in good alignment for each exercise, continue the set each day for 40 days as you master the mental poise and meditation of the full set.

Kriya for Lower Spine and Elimination

1. Sit up straight with the legs stretched out. Bring the left leg under the buttocks so you **sit on the left heel**. Place both hands palm down next to the hips. Inhale deeply. As you exhale bend forward. Inhale— come back up. Continue for **2 minutes**.

2. Sit up straight and **extend both legs forward**. With the palms beside the hips, inhale deeply and exhale, bending forward, bringing the nose toward the knees. Continue for **2 minutes**.

3. a) Lie down on the back. Inhale deeply. b) As you exhale, sit up, grasp the toes, and bend forward. Inhale and lie down again. Mentally vibrate *Sat* on the inhale, *Nam* on the exhale. Continue with deep breaths for **2 minutes**.

4. **Plow Pose and Forward Bend**: Begin by resting on your back. Raise the legs slowly up until the feet touch the ground over the head then let the legs back down. Sit up and grasp the toes. Continue alternating between the two postures, moving smoothly and continuously for **2 minutes**.

5. Lie down on the back. a) Bring the knees into the chest and press them close with your hands. b) Then, extend the legs straight. c) Sit up bending forward into Forward Bend, grasping the toes. Continue this cycle rhythmically for **2 minutes**.

6. Bend forward and grasp the toes with the legs out straight. **Do not let go of the toes** as you roll back on your spine into Plow Pose. Roll back and forth without letting go of the toes. Continue for **2 minutes**.

7. Relax completely.

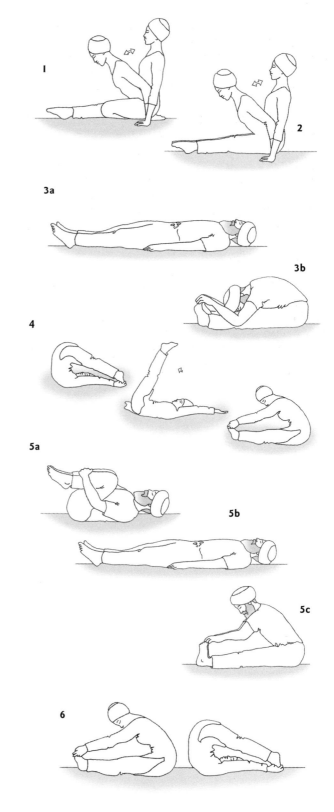

Comments:

The First, Second and Third Chakras associated with the rectum, sex organs and Navel Point are thoroughly exercised in this kriya. It gives flexibility of the spine and improves the power of digestion and elimination of waste and toxins. This is not a beginner's set; you need some flexibility to do it well.

riya for Nerve, Navel, & Lower Spine Strength

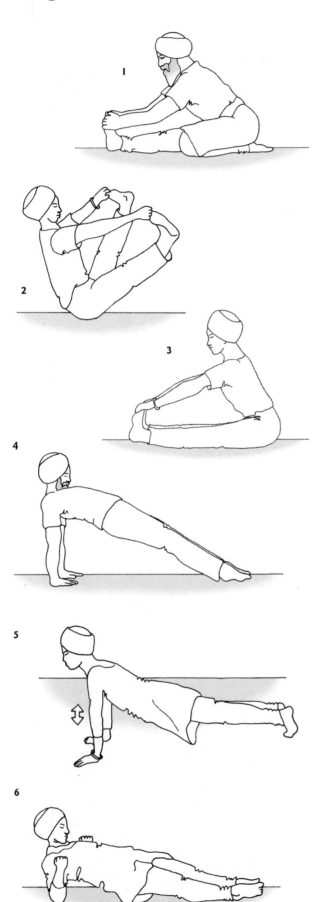

1. Sit with the left heel at the rectum and the right leg extended. Bend forward and grasp the toes with both hands. Straighten the spine and focus your eyes on the toes. Stay perfectly still with normal breathing and a light *mulbandh* applied. Continue for **3 minutes**. To end: Inhale deeply and pull back on the toes. Completely exhale, pull back more and apply a strong *mulbandh*. Repeat twice more. Relax.

2. **Kundalini Lotus**: Balance on the sacrum, grasp the toes of both feet and extend the legs up and wide at 60°. Keeping the spine straight, **apply a constant *mulbandh***. Breathe naturally. Hold for **3 minutes**. To end: Inhale deeply, exhale and apply a strong *mulbandh*. Repeat twice more and relax.

3. Extend both legs straight. Reach forward and hold onto the toes. Pull the spine up straight by pulling back on the toes. Apply a strong Chin Lock. Begin Long Deep Breathing. Continue for **3 minutes**. To end: Inhale, exhale and apply a strong *mulbandh*. Repeat twice more.

4. **Back Platform Pose**: With the legs extended straight, put the palms on the ground behind you with the fingertips pointing towards the toes. Lift the chest and buttocks up until the body is straight with only the heels and palms on the ground. Bring the chin to the chest. Press the toes forward. Breathe naturally. Continue for **3 minutes**. To end: Inhale deeply, exhale and apply *mulbandh*. Repeat twice more and relax.

5. Lie on the stomach. Put the palms on the ground under the shoulders. **Push up** off the ground with the body straight until you form a **front platform**. Exhale as you slowly go down to the ground. Inhale as you slowly rise up. Do not apply *mulbandh*. Continue with deep, slow breaths **26 times**. Relax.

6. Lie on the back. Rise up on the elbows; the elbows are aligned beneath the shoulders. Raise the buttocks up so the spine and body are straight. Chin is tucked. Only the heels and elbows are on the ground. Point the toes. Hold the pose with **Long Deep Breathing**. Continue for **3 minutes**. Inhale, then exhale completely and apply *mulbandh*.

Comments:

This kriya is a good physical workout that requires flexibility and endurance and some familiarity with the basics of Kundalini Yoga exercise. The lower nerve plexuses are pressured and the vital energy is raised above the diaphragm. If you experience chronic

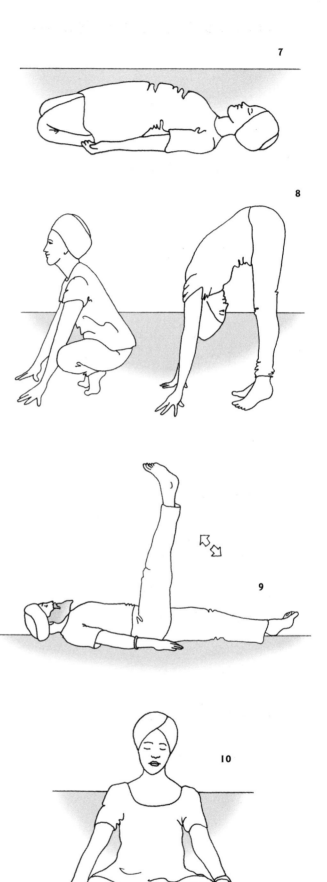

7. Sit on the heels. Slowly lean back until the head and possibly the shoulders are on the ground. The arms are relaxed on the ground beside the legs. Keep a light, constant *mulbandh* applied. Begin **Long Deep Breathing**. Continue for **3 minutes**. To end: Inhale, exhale completely, and apply a strong *mulbandh*. Repeat twice more. Relax.

8. **Frog Pose**: squat down with the knees wide and the fingertips on the ground between the knees; the heels are together and lifted. Inhale—raise the buttocks up as the head drops; keep the heels lifted and pressed together. Exhale—return to the original position with the head lifted. Continue with deep breaths. 30 repetitions.

9. **Alternate Leg Lifts**: Lie on the back. Place the arms relaxed along the sides of the body with the palms down. Inhale—lift one leg up to 90°. Exhale—let it down smoothly to the ground. Switch legs with each breath cycle. On the inhale, apply a slight *mulbandh*. Continue for **3 minutes**.

10. Sit in a comfortable meditation posture. Pull in the Navel Point and apply *mulbandh*. Mentally view the entire body. Scan through each area and every cell systematically. As you do this your mind will send many thoughts. The thoughts will be whatever is associated with the feelings and memories stored in that area of the body. The subconscious will also release thoughts. Reject any thought. Do not agree to the identification they invite. Free the body and cells to be neutral, present and faithful only to your consciousness. Whether the thoughts are true or false does not matter. Simply assert your presence to be as you are and nothing else. If the thought is "I am sitting," think "I am not sitting." If it is "I am not sitting," reject that as well and just be. Let all thoughts release and resolve themselves into the vastness of your being that includes all polarities. Each thought naturally invites you to action or identification. Stay neutral. You are not the body, mind, or spirit but the consciousness that gives rise to and integrates them all. Continue at least 3 minutes.

constipation or digestive problems, this set is of great value. If you want to stay steady under tense situations, this set is excellent. It frees your body from past patterns and opens you to the creative possibilities in the present moment.

Reserve Energy Set

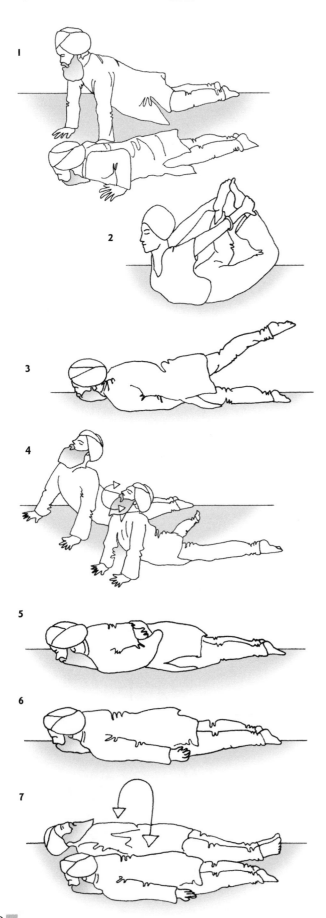

1. Lie on the stomach, heels together, tops of the feet remain on the floor. Inhale—rise up to a push-up position. Exhale down. Continue **15 repetitions** in a moderately slow rhythm.

2. **Bow Pose**: Still on the stomach, reach back and grab the ankles, stretching up. Begin **Breath of Fire** for **30 seconds**. Inhale, exhale, and relax on the stomach.

3. Still on the stomach. Place the chin on the floor and make fists of the hands and place them beneath you—just in front of the pelvis, at the bend in the leg. Inhale—raise the left leg up. Exhale—raise the right leg as the left leg is lowered. Continue alternating the legs with the breath. **2 minutes**.

4. **Cobra Pose**: Lift up the chest, arch the head back, keep the heels together and straighten the arms. Relax in this posture 45 seconds. Now spread the legs wide and bring the hands closer to the body to create a deeper arch in the back. With the chin lifted, turn the head from left to right. Inhale to the right and exhale to the left. Continue for 4-5 breaths.

5. Relax and lie down on the stomach. Grab the wrists behind the back and roll left and right on the chest, keeping the legs straight and the heels together. 30 seconds.

6. Still on the stomach, relax the arms down by the sides. Begin relaxing each part of the body. **Go deeply within yourself. 5 minutes.**

7. **Bundle Roll**: Lie straight on the back with the arms stiff at your sides. Roll from your stomach to your back and from your back to your stomach—flipping back and forth—without bending the body, arms, or legs. **Do not bend anywhere. 3 minutes**.

8. **Corpse Pose**: Deep relaxation on the back. 10 minutes.

Comments:

To tap the reserve flow of the kundalini energy in your body, you activate the sexual energy in Exercise 1, the navel energy in 2 and 3, and move that energy up the spine in exercise 4. During Exercise 4, the thyroid gland is stimulated and opens circulation to the upper brain as the head turns left and right. This clears your thinking and adds energy to the will. The last two exercises charge and strengthen your electromagnetic field and stabilize the new energy state you have created. This set gives you an extra resistance to the fluctuations of the environment.

Come into a lunge with the right foot forward and the left foot stretched back behind you, with the top of the foot on the ground. Extend the arms forward, parallel to the ground, with the palms together. Tilt the spine slightly forward of the vertical position. **Fix the eyes on the horizon or at the Brow Point**.

Take a deep breath and begin a rhythmic chant of **Sat Nam.** Emphasize the sound **Sat** as you pull the Navel Point in and apply a light *mulbandh*. Continue for 90 seconds. Then inhale. Relax.

Switch and place the left leg forward and right leg back. Repeat the exercise for an equal period of time.

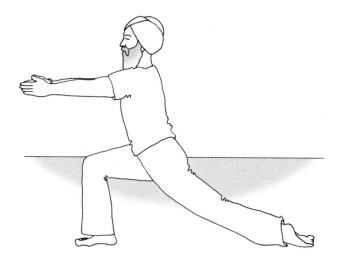

Comments:

This kriya will make you sweat if you do it properly. You may also notice a burning sensation in the cheeks. The time of practice can slowly be increased to 7½ minutes on each side. The practice and perfection of this kriya is said to optimize the responsiveness of the pituitary secretion, regulate excessive sexual energy, and increase general immunity to disease. It tests the nerve strength and balances the magnetic field of the body. If you don't want to be shaky when you are older, this is an excellent practice to start when you are young. Besides practicing this kriya by itself, it is enjoyable to do it after completing a long series of exercises that have worked on flexibility and circulation. The kriya helps transform the 'vital juices,' the *ojas*, into a form that can be used to maintain your entire nervous system.

Kriya for Conquering Sleep

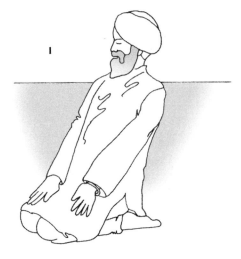

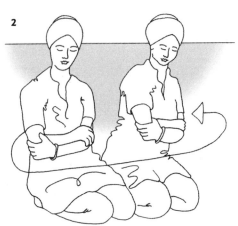

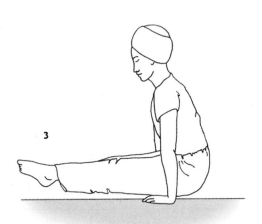

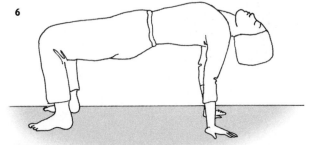

1. Sit on the heels with the palms on the thighs. Keep the spine straight and **lean back 30°** from vertical. Hold the posture with **Long Deep Breathing for 1 minute**. Relax.

2. Still sitting on the heels, fold the arms across the chest and hold onto the elbows. Rotate the torso in a circle from right to left (counterclockwise). Continue this grinding motion for **3 minutes**.

3. **Body Drops**: Immediately extend the legs in front of you. Put the hands on the ground next to the hips. With the inhale lift the hips and the heels off the ground. With the exhale drop the body. Complete **20 body drops**.

4. **Repeat Exercise 2** for 3 minutes.

5. Do **15 body drops**.

6. **Bridge Pose**: Sit with the knees bent and the hands, palms flat slightly behind the hips. Feet are flat on the ground about two fists apart. Press the hips up and let the head relax back. Hold the pose for **1 minute** with **normal breathing**. Continue with **Breath of Fire** for **3 minutes**. Inhale, exhale completely, and hold the breath out as you apply *mulbandh*. Inhale and relax.

7. Do **10 body drops**.

8. Repeat **Bridge Pose** for **3 minutes** with **Breath of Fire**.

Comments:

If deep, uninterrupted sleep is a frequent problem for you, practice this kriya regularly for 90 days. It can be done before bed at night or in the morning. A restful, rejuvenating sleep is very important to your health, to your emotional balance and for your memory

9. Relax completely on the back for 2 or 3 minutes.

10. Come into **Bridge Pose** and raise the right leg 60°. Point the toes forward. Begin a powerful **Breath of Fire** for **90 seconds**. Then inhale deeply, exhale completely, and apply *mulbandh*. **Repeat the exercise** with the left leg raised. Relax.

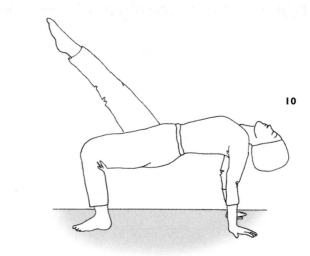

10

11. **Crow Pose**: Squat with the feet flat on the ground. Extend the arms in front parallel to the ground with the palms facing down. Inhale deeply and stand up—exhale completely as you squat down. Keep the spine as straight as possible. **30 repetitions**.

12. **Cobra Pose**: Hold the pose with normal breathing for 1 minute. Then kick the buttocks with one heel for **2 minutes**. Each time the heel strikes the buttocks, exhale slightly. Then kick with the other heel for **2 more minutes**. Relax.

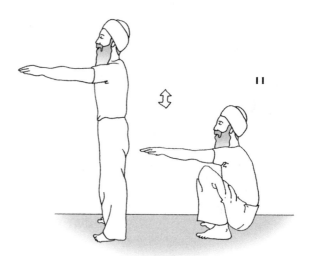

11

13. Sit on the heels in Rock Pose. Extend the arms straight over the head with the palms flat together. Bring the mudra halfway down toward the top of the head so that the elbows are slightly bent. Raise the eyes up and focus at the center of the skull on the pineal gland and project through the crown of the head. Continue for **3 minutes** or more.

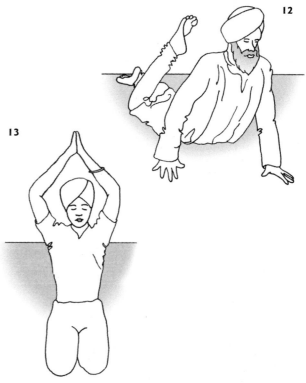

12

13

capacity. This natural approach takes some consistent effort but it has sure results and no unwanted side-effects. If you choose to put the effort into this kriya, it will eliminate many common sleep disturbances and give you alertness throughout the day.

Abdominal Strengthening

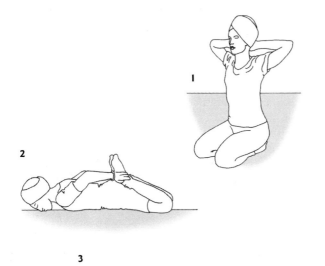

1. Sit on the heels in **Rock Pose**. Interlace the fingers behind the neck—**Venus Lock**. Spread the elbows wide apart. Begin **Breath of Fire** for **2 minutes**.

2. Lie on the stomach. Reach back and grab the ankles. Pull the ankles toward the buttocks keeping the chest on the ground. Hold for **2 minutes**.

3. **Stretch Pose**: Lie on the back. Raise the head and heels six inches off the ground. Point the hands toward the toes. Begin **Breath of Fire** for **2 minutes**.

4. Lie on the back. Begin a piston motion with the legs keeping them parallel to the ground. Breathe deeply. Continue for **2 minutes**.

5. Still on the back, keep the legs together with the toes pointed forward. Inhale and smoothly raise both legs to 90°. Then exhale as you lower them. Breathe deeply. Continue for **2 minutes**.

6. Lie on the stomach. Place the palms on the ground under the shoulders. Slowly arch up into Cobra Pose. Now lift the feet up toward the head and hold for **2 minutes**.

7. Lie on the back. Hug the knees into the chest and rock forward and back on the spine. Continue for **2 minutes**.

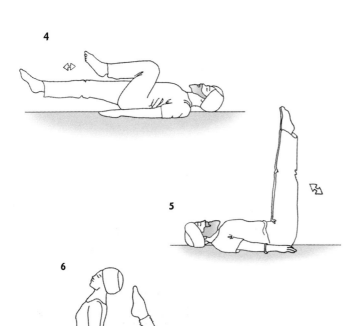

Comments:

This kriya gives you a good physical workout. It strengthens the navel point, abdominal muscles, and lower back. It improves circulation. It strengthens the nervous system so that your behavior can be constant and direct. It is an excellent set for strengthening the digestive system.

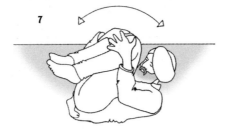

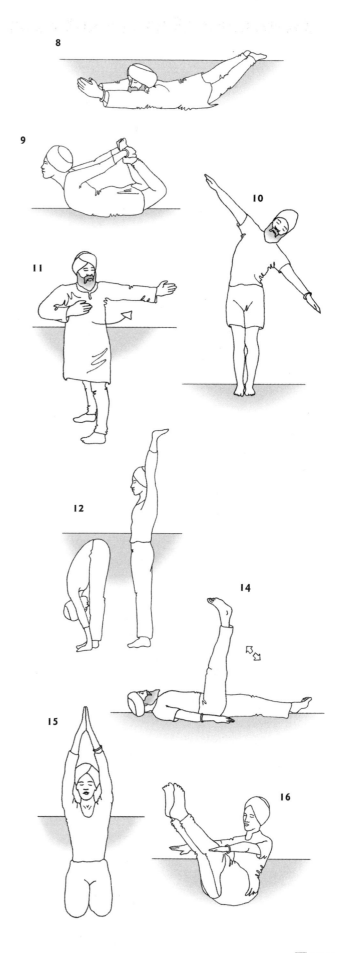

8. **Locust Pose**: Lie on the stomach. Extend the arms forward with the palms flat together. Lift the arms, chest and legs of the ground, arching the spine. Hold this extended locust with **Breath of Fire** for **2 minutes**.

9. **Bow Pose**: Still on the stomach, reach back and grasp the ankles. Arch up, lifting the chest and thighs off the ground and begin **Breath of Fire** for **2 minutes**, then relax.

10. **Side Stretch**: Stand up straight. Keep the legs together. Extend the arms to the sides, parallel to the ground with palms facing down. Without twisting the torso, bend to the left with a deep inhale, then bend to the right with the exhale. Continue this pendulum-like motion for **2 minutes**.

11. Still standing with the arms spread wide, spread the legs about two feet apart and turn the palms to the front. Inhale and stretch the left arm back parallel to the ground as the right hand comes to the Heart Center; exhale as the right arms stretches back parallel to the ground and the left hand comes to the Heart Center. Continue alternating from side to side for **2 minutes**.

12. Still standing, inhale and raise both arms straight up with wrists extended and the palms facing up; exhale as you bend forward and try to put the palms on the ground. Continue, alternating with the breath, for **2 minutes**.

13. Repeat Exercise 4. Breathe deeply. 2 minutes.

14. **Alternate Leg Lifts**: On your back, inhale and lift the left leg to 90°. Exhale as you lower it. Repeat with the right leg. Breathe deeply. **2 minutes**.

15. **Sat Kriya** with palms in **Prayer Pose** above the head. Sit on the heels with the arms stretched up and the palms together. Men cross the right thumb over the left; women cross left thumb over right. Pull in the Navel Point and say *Sat*, relax the Navel Point and say *Nam*. Continue rhythmically for **2 minutes**. Then inhale deeply, hold, apply *mulbandh*. Relax.

16. **Boat Pose**: Sit straight with the legs extended. Lift the legs up 60° from the ground. Extend the arms parallel to the ground with the palms down. Begin **Breath of Fire**. Continue for **2 minutes**. Then totally relax.

Flexibility and the Spine

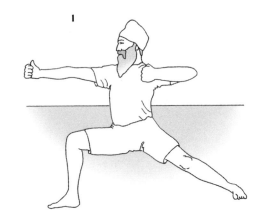

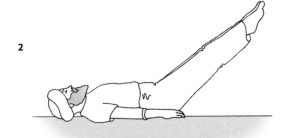

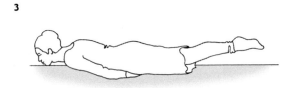

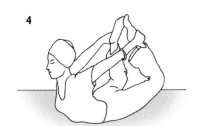

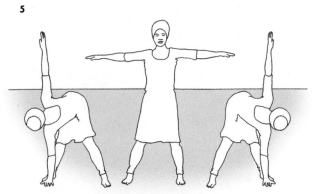

1. **Archer Pose**: Stand with the right leg bent forward so the knee is over the toes. The left leg is straight back with the foot flat on the ground at a 45° angle; align the center of the arch of the left foot with the heel of the right. Raise the right arm straight in front, parallel to the ground and make a fist as if grasping a bow. Pull the left arm back as if pulling the bowstring back to the shoulder. Feel a stretch across the chest and tension between the shoulder blades. The head is turned so that the gaze is fixed on the horizon, beyond the right fist. Hold the position **3–5 minutes**, then **switch legs** and arms and **repeat**.

2. Immediately lie on the back. Put the heels together and lift both legs two feet from the ground. Hold the position **1–3 minutes** with **Long Deep Breathing**.

3. **Locust Pose**: Lie down on the stomach. Make fists with the hands and put them beneath you–just in front of the pelvis, at the bend in the leg. Keeping the heels together and the legs straight, lift them up as high as possible and hold this position for **3 minutes**.

4. **Bow Pose**: Still on the stomach, reach back and firmly grasp the ankles. Lift the chest and the thighs, arching the back up from the ground. Hold the position for **2–3 minutes**.

5. Stand up straight and spread the legs two feet apart. Touch the right hand to the floor in front of the left foot. The left arm is pointing back. Switch sides and continue this alternate motion with long breaths. On the inhale, rise up completely; on the exhale touch the toe. Repeat **25 times on each side**.

6. Stand up with the legs 6 inches apart. On the exhale, bend forward and place the palms flat on the ground. Inhale and rise up stretching backwards with the arms over the head. Continue **25 times**.

7. Stand with the legs 6 inches apart. Bend to the side stretching the opposite arm over the head. Alternate smoothly from side to side; inhaling as you stretch, exhaling as you come up. Keep the chest square; do not let the torso bend forward or backward. Continue **25 times on each side**.

8. **Life Nerve Stretch**: Sit down and spread the legs wide. Grab the big toe of each foot by locking the forefingers around the toe, pressing the thumb into the toenail. Keeping a firm grip, inhale and arch the spine up straight; exhale and touch the head to the right knee. Inhale center and exhale down to the left knee. Continue alternating, **25 times on each side**. Inhale center, hold the breath and exhale to transition to the next posture.

9. **Forward Bend**: Bring the legs together while still holding onto the toes. Inhale and arch up, exhale and pull the head down to the knees. Continue this pumping motion **25 times**.

10. **Plow Pose**: Lie flat on the back. Slowly raise the legs over the head until they touch the floor. In this position, bring the arms over the head, fingertips pointing toward the toes. Keep the knees straight and flex the ankles so that the toes rest on the ground. Relax in this position for **5 minutes**. Then slowly lower the legs back down to the ground.

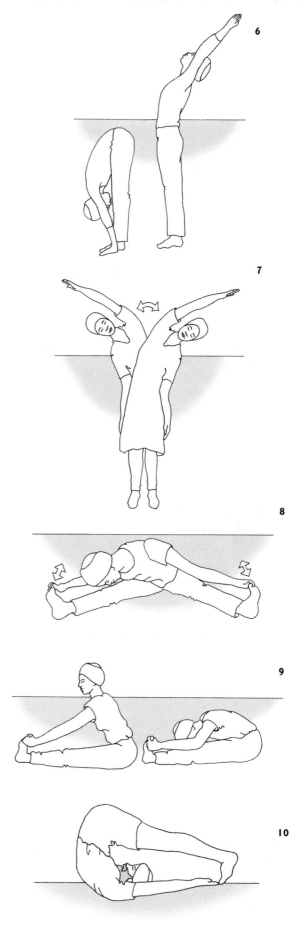

Continued on next page...

Flexibility and the Spine

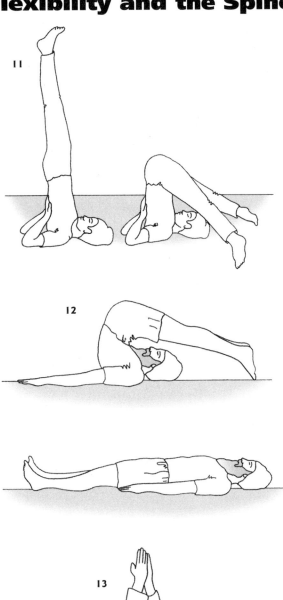

11. **Shoulder Stand**: Come into this position by raising the legs straight up toward the ceiling from Plow Pose. Support the spine perpendicular to the ground with the hands. Rest the weight on the elbows. Hold this position for **3–5 minutes**. Then bring the legs down into Plow Pose, with the legs spread wide. Slowly move from this position to Shoulder Stand 4 times. Lower the legs and spine and rest on the back.

12. Alternate from lying on the back to Plow Pose, keeping the arms in their original position, palms down by the hips. Continue **50 times**. If necessary, the hands may be used to lift the legs up and back. Relax for 3 minutes.

13. **Sat Kriya**: Sit on the heels with the arms overhead and the palms together. Interlace the fingers except for the index fingers, which point straight up. Men cross the right thumb over the left with the left little finger is on the bottom; women cross left thumb over right, right pinkie on bottom. Chant *Sat* and pull the Navel Point in; chant *Nam* and release it. Continue powerfully with a steady rhythm for **5 minutes**. Inhale and draw the energy up the spine to the Brow Point. Exhale and immediately transition to the next posture.

14. Bend forward into Gurpranam: Place the forehead on the ground and stretch the arms overhead on the floor, keeping the palms together. Meditate at the Brow Point by silently projecting the primal sounds, **Sa Ta Na Ma**. Continue for **31 minutes**.

Comments:

This set is an example of a series which would not be given in a beginner's Kundalini Yoga class. It is for students who have attained a moderate degree of flexibility and coordination in regular classes and sadhana, and who want to eject residual poisons and drugs from the muscle tissue. If the set is done every morning for six months, it adjusts the spine very well. Before attempting this set, with guidance from a Kundalini Yoga instructor, be sure you have no major

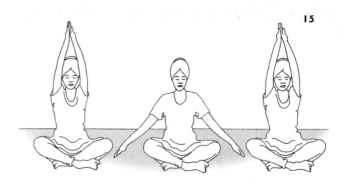

15. Sit in **Easy Pose**. Inhale and raise both arms overhead bringing the backs of the hands together. Exhale and lower the arms letting just the fingertips touch the floor. Continue for 5 minutes.

16. Stand up and extend the arms out in front of you, parallel to the ground. Begin **25 deep knee bends** into Crow Pose, keeping the spine straight and the feet flat.

17. **Cat–Cow**: Rest on the hands and knees. a) Flex the spine and raise your head on the inhale; b) on the exhale, extend the spine, arching it up as you lower your head. Continue for **5 minutes**.

18. Deeply relax for **15–30 minutes on your back**. This is a vigorous set. You will sweat; so cover yourself up with a blanket to keep from getting cold.

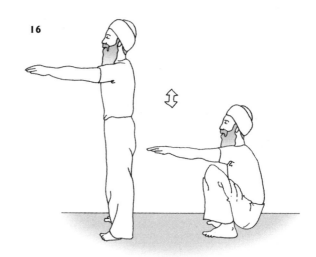

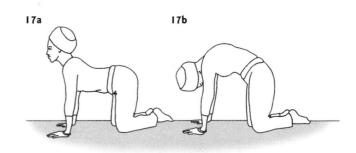

physical problem that will prevent you from doing any of the exercises.

Unlike most Kundalini Yoga kriyas, you do not take a 2–3 minute rest between each exercise unless it is explicitly stated. The set can be adapted to a regular class by limiting the times of the exercises to 1–2 minutes and by adding rest periods between the different postures.

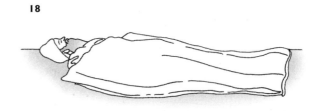

Sex Energy Transformation

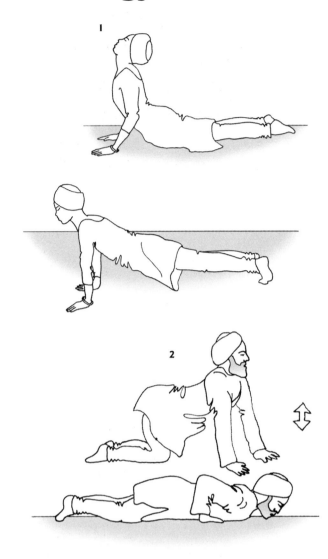

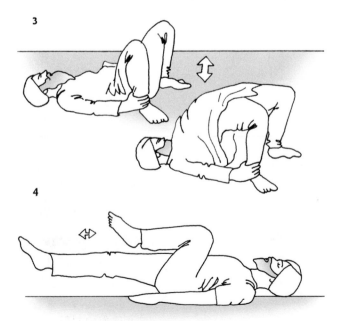

1. Lie on the stomach. Place the hands on the ground directly under the shoulders. Lift up into **Cobra Pose** with the head arching back. Inhale and raise the hips straight off the ground coming into a **Front Platform Pose**. Exhale as you lower the hips to the ground and come back into Cobra Pose Repeat **26 times**, then relax on the stomach for 2 minutes.

   Note to the teacher: Chant "Ong"—the Infinite, creative consciousness, on the inhale; and "Sohung"—I am Thou, on the exhale. This will keep a rhythm and keep the mind focused.

2. Come into Cow Pose and inhale. Stretch forward on the exhale, allowing the hips and the chin to touch the ground. Keep the head up and the arms bent. Inhale back into Cow Pose.

   Note to the teacher: Continue to chant "Ong–Sohung": "Ong" on the forward motion, "Sohung" on resuming Cow Pose. Repeat **26 times**.

3. **Pelvic Lifts**: Immediately without resting, lie down on the back. Bend the knees and grasp the ankles with the hands. The soles of the feet should stay on the ground next to the buttocks. Inhale—lift the hips. Exhale—relax them down. Repeat **26 times**. **Rest for 2 minutes**. Repeat **26 more times**.

4. Immediately extend both legs and raise them 18 inches from the floor. Start Long Deep Breathing for 30 seconds. Breathe powerfully. Then begin a piston motion with the legs; bring one knee to the chest, then the other with each deep inhale. Continue alternating with this push-pull action for up to 1 minute. Inhale—extend both legs straight out for 5 seconds. Relax.

5. Lie on the back. Bring the soles of the feet together and grab them with the hands. Rock forward and back on the spine for 30–45 seconds.

6. Deep relaxation for 2 minutes.

7. **Stretch Pose**: Lift the feet and the head 6 inches off the ground with **normal breathing**. Focus the eyes on the toes. Balance in this position and hold it for **up to 7 minutes**. Inhale deeply, exhale, hold the breath out and apply *mulbandh*. Hold the breath out as long as possible. Repeat the inhale, exhale, *mulbandh*: 4 more times. Then relax down.

8. Completely **relax for 5 minutes** letting the energy circulate. Think of God and God-consciousness. Feel unlimited. After 5 minutes come back from relaxation by **chanting "God and me, me and God, are One"** about **12 times**, raising the pitch and volume smoothly across these repetitions. Inhale deeply, hold for 15 seconds, then exhale. Start the chant again but very powerfully. Chant loudly from the Navel Point and solar plexus. The eyes should be closed. **Do not feel shy**. To end: inhale and exhale eight times, then inhale and suspend the breath and raise the legs to 90°; hold for 15 seconds. Exhale and relax.

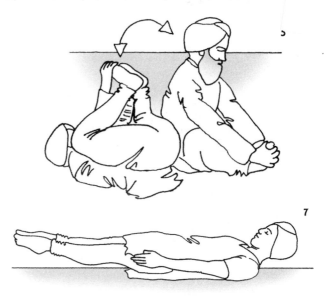

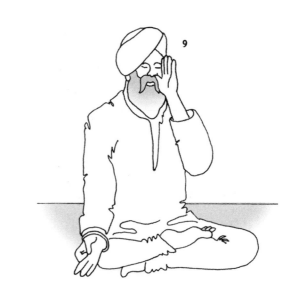

9. Sit in Sidhasana (Perfect Pose), or Sukasana (Easy Pose). Use the thumb and little finger of one hand to close alternate nostrils. There should be **no break between the sequence of pranayam**—each flows into the next.
a. Inhale through the left nostril, exhale through the right. Meditate at the base of the spine and pull *mulbandh*. On the inhale, think *Sat*; on the exhale vibrate *Nam*. Continue for 1 minute.
b. Breath of Fire: inhale through the left nostril, exhale through the right for 1 minute.
c. Inhale and exhale through the left nostril only, moderately fast for about 15 seconds.
d. Begin Breath of Fire through the left nostril for 15 seconds, then through the right nostril for 15 seconds. Then again through the left nostril for 5 seconds and through the right for 5 seconds.

To end: Release the hand and inhale through both nostrils and hold 5 seconds. Exhale, holding the breath out for the next 30 seconds. As you suspend the breath out flow smoothly through this visualization: mentally repeat *Sat Nam*, visualize the sound following an upward spiral along the spine. Then visualize *Sat* going down both sides of the spine, entering the base of the spine and *Nam* rising up the middle of the spine. Close the mind to every other thing and concentrate. Now is the time. One or two more times, inhale deeply and exhale then repeat the mental visualization.

Continued next page...

Sex Energy Transformation

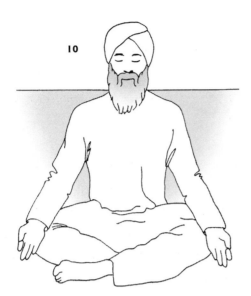

10

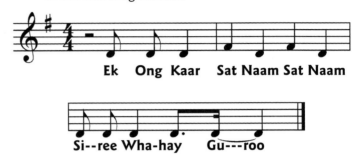

10. Chant *Ek Ong Kar Sat Nam Sat Nam Siri Wahe Guru* in the following manner:

Ek   Ong   Kaar   Sat Naam Sat Naam

Si--ree Wha-hay   Gu---roo

When chanting *Sat Nam* and *Guru*, apply and release *mulbandh*. Gradually the *mulbandh* will become so strong and locked that it will be easy to hold throughout the entire chant. Continue chanting for **6 minutes**. To end: Inhale—hold for 15 seconds. Exhale and relax or meditate.

Comments:

In our culture, we are taught to view sex in terms of pleasure and reproduction. We are not taught the need for moderation in sex in order to maintain our health and nerve balance. Sexual experience in the correct consciousness can give you the experience of God and bliss, but before that can ever occur you must charge your sexual batteries and nurture real potency. The seminal fluids produced in the male and the fluids produced in the female contain high concentrations of minerals and elements that are crucial to proper nerve balance and brain functioning. According to the yoga tradition, these sexual fluids, or *ojas*, are reabsorbed by the body if allowed to mature and the minerals and nutrient elements are taken into the spinal fluid. Running your brain without the *ojas* is like running a car without oil—you wear out quickly. It was said that the main use of the sexual energy was to repair and rejuvenate the organs of the body. If the body is well cared

for and nutrition is well-balanced, the yogi maintains potency and sexual interest throughout the lifespan. Usually we see potency waning as early as the 40s. This kriya will generate sexual energy and transmute it into *ojas for healing and continued sexual vitality.* The first three exercises activate the Second Chakra; then the Navel Point and lower spine. Exercise 3 is especially effective for relieving tension and problems of the ovaries. Exercise 4 and 5 move the energy out of the digestive system. Exercise 7 distributes the energy from the Navel Point above the solar plexus to the Heart Center. Exercise 9 uses pranayam to completely open your psychic channels and move the kundalini energy all the way to the highest chakras. Exercise 10 uses the kundalini energy in the mantra to project the mind into the infinity of the cosmos and beyond our normal earthly consciousness.

Prayer is when the mind is one-pointed and man talks to Infinity. Meditation is when the mind becomes totally clean and receptive and Infinity talks to man. That is what meditation is.

There are two levels of meditation. In one, this unit self talks to Infinity. In the other, Infinity talks to the unit. All the other stages are preparations for meditation. . . . The best way to meditate is in a creative meditation. The logic behind this is that the mind is mostly tuned to the intellect. The intellect starts giving thoughts and more thoughts, which relate to your emotion and temperament. They become desire, and desire then directs the body to create a creativity to earn the object or goal. This creativity is a practical experience in life. . . . You can't live without meditation. Imagination and activity get blended to affect the focusing of the personality. That's what meditation is. You relate your unit activity toward your word of Infinity. The question is: Are you creative or uncreative? That will decide the trend of your life.

If you just sit for twenty minutes and close yourself, that's not meditation. . . . Meditation is the creativity and activity which relates your existence to the existence of the cosmos. It is individual harmony in relationship to universal harmony.

Laya Yoga Meditation

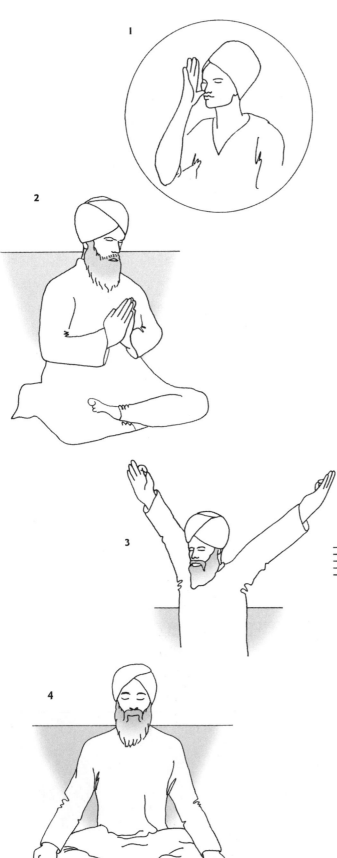

1. Sit in Easy Pose with a straight spine. Block off the right nostril with your right thumb. Begin deep breathing through the left nostril. Close the eyes and survey the body up and down. Complete **10 deep breaths through the left nostril**. Change hands and continue with **10 deep breaths through the right nostril**.

2. Bring the hands to Prayer Pose at the center of the chest. Press the palms firmly together and the sides of the thumbs steadily against the chest. Begin **Long Deep Breathing for 2 minutes**; then **Breath of Fire** for **1 minute**.

3. Bring the arms to 60° with the hands in Gyan Mudra, palms facing each other. Begin **Long Deep Breathing** for **2 minutes**.

4. Keeping the hands in Gyan Mudra, lower the arms, resting the wrists on the knees with the elbows straight. Begin the 3½–cycle Laya Yoga chant, pulling *mulbandh*. With the breath, spin the sound current up the spine. Let go and get lost in the spin. Visualize the sound spinning from the base of the spine to the top of the head. Use the Adi Shakti Mantra, shown here phonetically: Ek Ong Kaar-(uh), Sat-a Naam-(uh), Siree Wha-(uh) Hay Guroo. On "Ek," pull the Navel Point. With each "uh," pull the diaphragm lock (uddiyana bandh) successively higher and tighter. On "Hay Guroo" relax the lock. Continue for **11 to 31 minutes**.

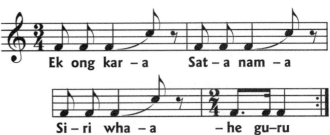

Ek ong kar – a   Sat – a nam – a

Si – ri wha – a   – he gu–ru

Comments:

There are two voices within us: One is the voice of the ego and the other, the voice of the soul. Justify yourself before the Creator, not before others. Consciously remember the link between you and your Creator. If you can stay free of entanglement from negativity, you are a living god on this earth. This meditation enables one to get lost in the sound current. "Meditate and feel God for 40 days and you will be liberated."

Seven-Wave "Sat Nam" Meditation

Sit in Easy Pose. Bring the hands to Prayer Pose at the center of the chest, thumbs touching the center of the sternum. With the eyes closed, look up slightly, focusing at the Brow Point. Inhale deeply, concentrating on the breath. With the exhale, chant the mantra in the "law of seven" or "law of the tides." Vibrate *Sat* in six waves, and let *Nam* be the seventh wave

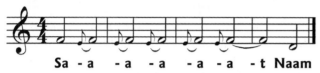

Sa - a - a - a - a - t Naam

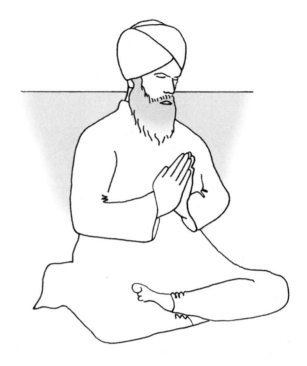

On each wave, thread the sound through the chakras beginning at the base of the spine, the First Chakra. On *Nam*, let the energy and sound radiate out from the Seventh Chakra at the crown of the head through the aura. As the sound penetrates each chakra, or center, gently pull the physical area it corresponds to. The first center is the rectum, the second is the sex organs, the third is the Navel Point, the fourth is the heart, the fifth is the throat, the sixth is the Brow Point and the seventh is the top of the head. Continue for **15 minutes**.

Comments:

If you can build this meditation to at least 31 minutes 6 seconds per day, the mind will be cleansed as the ocean waves wash the sandy beach.

This is a *bij* (seed) mantra meditation. *Bij* mantras such as *Sat Nam* are the only sounds which can totally rearrange the habit patterns of the subconscious mind. We all have habit patterns. We could not function without them, but sometimes the patterns we have created are not wanted. You have changed, so you want the patterns to change. By vibrating the sound current *Sat Nam* in this manner, you activate the energy of the mind that erases and establishes habits. Consequently, this meditation is good to do as an introduction to Kundalini Yoga. It will open the mind to new experiences. A long-time student will still meditate in this way, particularly to clear off the effects of a hurried day before beginning another deep meditation. After you chant this mantra, you will feel calm and relaxed.

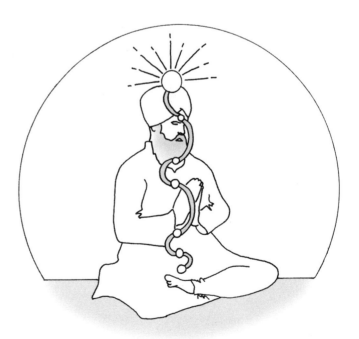

Raj Yoga Meditation with Maha Bandh

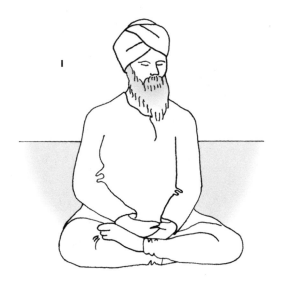

Men

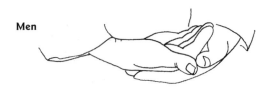

Women

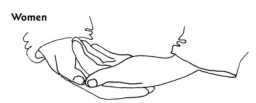

1. Sit in any easy sitting posture. The spine must be perfectly straight. Rest both hands palms up, gently in the lap. Women rest the left hand on top of the right; men reverse the hands. Close the eyes and concentrate at the Brow Point. Bring your awareness to the tip of the big toe and mentally draw the life force along the entire length of the leg to the rectum and rotate the energy around the ring of the rectum. Inhale deeply—pull the rectum up (*mulbandh*) and release it. Continue rhythmically pulling *mulbandh* and then exhale. **Repeat the cycle, inhaling from toe to rectum. 5 minutes. Continue visualizing from the toe—drawing the energy from the earth to the base—and further up with each exercise.**

2. Inhale and pull the sex organ as well as the rectum. Contract it and pull up 5 times per breath. **5 minutes**.

3. Pull the Navel Point, sex organ and rectum five times per breath. Try to massage the spine with the Navel Point. Pull the lower triangle further up each time until the energy is pulled all the way to the diaphragm. **5 minutes**.

4. Inhale deeply and concentrate on the Divine Power in the breath. Feel it shoot up to the diaphragm like a rocket as the locks are pulled. Lift up the chest and lift the diaphragm. Exhale and continue. **5 minutes**.

5. Inhale—pull all the locks and pull the chin in to form the Neck Lock, or *jalandhar bandh*, concentrate on consciously raising the energy to the neck. You may experience heat in the throat and neck. **5 minutes**.

Comments:

The timing for Exercise 7, the final meditation, is unspecified and may be as long as you want. The chanting of "Lah" may be extended to 11 minutes. It is best to practice this meditation 31 minutes to 1 hour each day.

Raj Yoga is a part of Kundalini Yoga. There are many meditations in this part of the tradition. This meditation awakens the God in you. There is no need to find God. It already exists in you as Infinite Awareness, ready to be awakened. This meditation

6. Inhale—pull the energy all the way to the Brow Point. Apply all the lower locks and press the eyes up. Exhale and continue. **5 minutes**.

7. Relax, meditate at the Brow Point, and go deep within.

8. With the eyes at the Brow Point, chant very sweetly from the back of your throat at the upper palate of the mouth. Open your mouth and your throat to create the sound.

La-a-a-a-a-a-a-ah

Create a continuous sound, inhaling when necessary. Listen to the sound as though it comes from Infinity. After **5 minutes**, inhale deeply. Tilt the head back and look at the sky. Let the breath out with a laugh. Keep **laughing aloud for 30 seconds**. Relax.

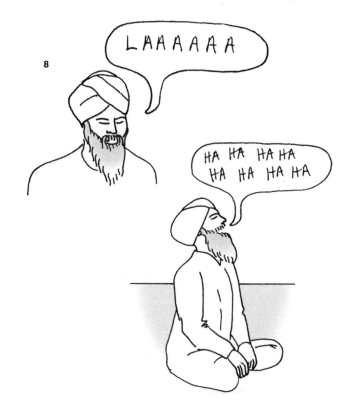

can open the Third Eye and give you the practical experience of a reality which cannot be put into words. Raj Yoga relates the mind directly to the soul or self. There is no automatic control over the mind except will. Kundalini Yoga generally relates the body directly to soul so that the mind has no option but to follow the will to Infinity.

This series will automatically relate your circumvent force to the universal magnetic field. The more you consciously invest your mind into this, the more expansion you will experience.

Kirtan Kriya

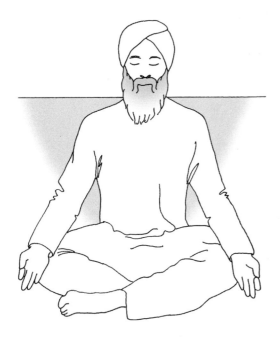

This kriya is one of three that Yogi Bhajan mentioned would carry us through the Aquarian Age, even if all other teachings were lost. There are four principle components to practicing Kirtan Kriya correctly: Mantra, Mudra, Voice, and Visualization.

Mantra
This kriya uses the five primal sounds, or the *Panj Shabd*— S, T, N, M, A—in the original *bij* form of the word Sat Nam:

SA — infinity, cosmos, beginning
TA — life, existence
NA — death
MA — birth

This is the cycle of creation. From the Infinite comes life and individual existence. From life comes death or change. From death comes the rebirth of consciousness. From rebirth comes the joy of the Infinite through which compassion leads back to life. Chant the 'A' as if you were pronouncing 'mom,' in the following manner:

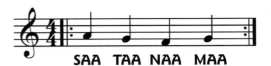

SAA TAA NAA MAA

Mudra
Each repetition of the entire mantra takes 3 to 4 seconds. The elbows are straight while chanting, and each finger touches, in turn, the tip of the thumb with a firm but gentle pressure.

Sa — the index or Jupiter finger touches the thumb;
Ta — the middle or Saturn finger and thumb;
Na — the ring or Sun finger and thumb;
Ma — the pinkie or Mercury finger and thumb; then begin again with the index finger.

Visualization
You must meditate on the primal sounds in the "L" form. This means that when you meditate you feel there is a constant inflow of cosmic energy into your solar center, or Tenth Gate (the Crown Chakra). As the energy enters the top of the head, you place **Sa**, **Ta**, **Na**, or **Ma** there.

As you chant **Sa**, for example, the "S" starts at the top of your head and the "A" moves down and out through the Brow Point, projected to Infinity. This energy flow follows the energy pathway called the golden cord—the connection between the pineal and pituitary gland. Some people may occasionally experience headaches from practicing Kirtan Kriya if they do not use this "L" form. The most common reason for this is improper circulation of prana in the solar centers.

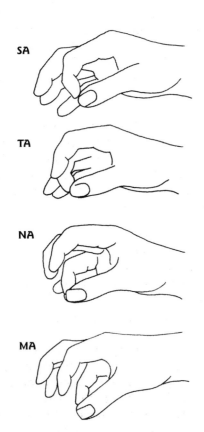

SA

TA

NA

MA

Voice

We chant the mantra in the three languages of consciousness:

Aloud	the voice of the human	awareness of the things of the world
Whisper	the voice of the lover	experiencing the longing to belong
Silent	the voice of the divine	meditate on Infinity or mentally vibrate

To Begin the Practice

Sit straight in Easy Pose and meditate at the Brow Point.

Chant aloud for 5 minutes, then whisper for 5 minutes and then go deeply into silence, mentally vibrating the sound. Vibrate in silence for 10 minutes, then whisper for 5 minutes, then chant aloud for 5 minutes.

Close the meditation with a deep inhale and suspend the breath as long as comfortable—up to a minute—relaxing it smoothly to complete 1 minute of absolute stillness and silence.

To end: Stretch the hands up as far as possible and spread the fingers wide. Stretch the spine and take several deep breaths. Relax.

Comments:

Each time you close a mudra by joining the thumb with a finger, your ego seals the effect of that mudra in your consciousness. The effects are as follows:

SIGN	FINGER	NAME	EFFECT
Jupiter	Index	Gyan Mudra	Knowledge
Saturn	Middle	Shuni Mudra	Wisdom, intelligence, patience
Sun	Ring	Surya Mudra	Vitality, energy of life
Mercury	Pinkie	Buddhi Mudra	Ability to communicate

Practicing this chant brings a total mental balance to the individual psyche. As you vibrate on each fingertip, you alternate your electrical polarities. The index and ring fingers are electrically negative, relative to the other fingers. This causes a balance in the electro-magnetic projection of the aura. If during the silent part of the meditation your mind wanders uncontrollably, go back to a whisper, to a loud voice, to a whisper and back into silence. Do this as often as necessary to stay alert.

Practicing this meditation is both a science and an art. It is an art in the way it molds consciousness and the refinement of sensation and insight it produces. It is a science in the tested certainty of the results it produces. Each meditation is based on the tested experience of many people, in many conditions, over many years. It is based on the structure of the psyche and the laws of action and reaction that accompany each sound, movement and posture. The meditations as kriyas code this science into specific formulas we can practice to get specific results. Because it is so effective and exact, it can also lead to problems if not done properly.

Chanting the *Panj Shabd*—the primal or nuclear form of *Sat Nam*—has profound energy within it because we are breaking the *bij* (seed or atom) of the sound, *Sat Nam*, into its primary elements. You may use this chant in any position as long as you adhere to the following requirements:

1. Keep the spine straight.
2. Focus at the Brow Point.
3. Use the "L" form of meditation.
4. Vibrate the *Panj Shabd* in all three languages—human, lover, and divine.
5. Use common sense without fanaticism.

The timing can be decreased or increased as long as you maintain the ratio of spoken, whispered, and silent chanting—always end with 1 minute of complete stillness and silence. Yogi Bhajan said, at the Winter Solstice of 1972, that a person who wears pure white and meditates on this sound current for 2½ hours a day for one year, will know the unknown and see the unseen. Through this constant practice, the mind awakens to the infinite capacity of the soul for sacrifice, service, and creation.

A Transcendental Meditation:
Maha Shakti Chalnee Indra Mudra

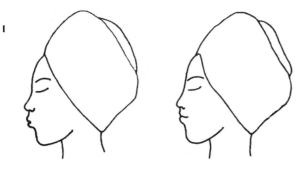

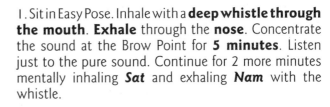

1. Sit in Easy Pose. Inhale with a **deep whistle through the mouth**. **Exhale** through the **nose**. Concentrate the sound at the Brow Point for **5 minutes**. Listen just to the pure sound. Continue for 2 more minutes mentally inhaling *Sat* and exhaling *Nam* with the whistle.

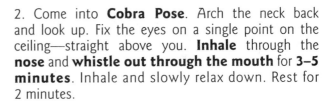

2. Come into **Cobra Pose**. Arch the neck back and look up. Fix the eyes on a single point on the ceiling—straight above you. **Inhale** through the **nose** and **whistle out through the mouth** for **3–5 minutes**. Inhale and slowly relax down. Rest for 2 minutes.

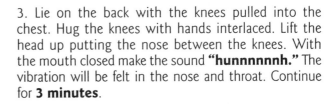

3. Lie on the back with the knees pulled into the chest. Hug the knees with hands interlaced. Lift the head up putting the nose between the knees. With the mouth closed make the sound **"hunnnnnnh."** The vibration will be felt in the nose and throat. Continue for **3 minutes**.

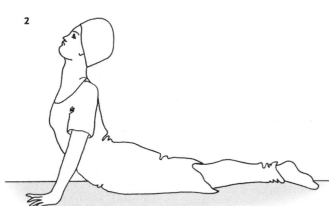

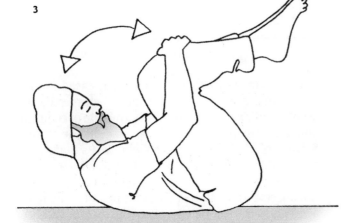

Comments:

This is a transcendental meditation as it was originally taught centuries ago. Transcendental meditations always have a breath rhythm and a hand mudra linked to the mantra. In the yogic scriptures, there are six pages written to tell the benefits of this single kriya. It allows you to control the senses and thoughts. It balances the *prana* and *apana vayus* (channels) to improve your health and increase your lung capacity. Once your lung capacity for normal breathing becomes greater than 700cc's, your personality changes. The extra capacity sends an increased vital force to the nervous system with each breath. Nerves that are strong give you patience.

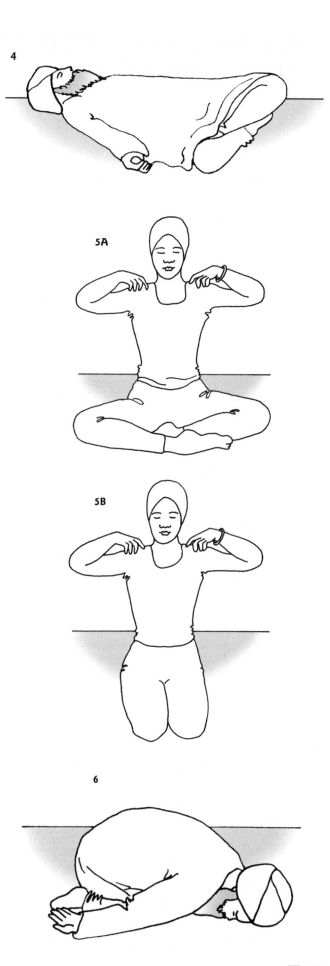

4. Relax on the back with legs crossed on the ground as in Easy Pose. This creates a delicate pressure in the lower spine. Maintain the position for **5 minutes**.

5. **Spinal Twist**: Sit up in Easy Pose, hands on the shoulders, thumbs behind and fingers in front. Swing from left to right, inhaling left and exhaling right. Synchronize the motion with the breath for **1 minute**, then **sit on the heels** and continue the exercise for **1 more minute**. Inhale, hold briefly, exhale.

6. **Baby Pose**: Still sitting on the heels, lean forward and put the forehead on the ground and allow your arms to rest back by the hips. Rest completely in this pose for **3–5 minutes**.

In this exercise, the body maintains a perfect equilibrium in the carbon dioxide and oxygen exchange. The pressure on the tongue causes the thyroid and parathyroid glands to secrete. If you practice Exercise 1 for 15 minutes, you may experience some pain in the ears. After 31 minutes, you may have a pain in the upper chest. These are the signs of the glands secreting and gaining a new balance. If you sincerely practiced Exercise 1 for 31 minutes a day followed by the remaining exercises, this kriya could change your personality, your total lifestyle, and even your destiny.

Heartbeat Meditation in the Triple Lock

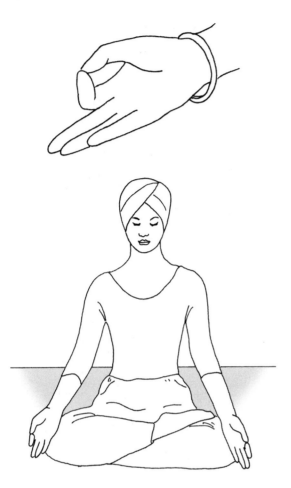

Sit in **Easy Pose** or Lotus Pose with the hands in **Gyan Mudra**, palms up, at the knees. Apply just enough pressure in the fingers (mudra) so that you clearly feel your pulse in the tips of the thumbs. The essence of this meditation is to form the triple lock in a relaxed, stable and attentive attitude. The triple lock is: 1) Gyan Mudra feeling your pulse, 2) front teeth locked on top of each other, tip to tip, lower jaw moving forward slightly from its natural position 3) tongue turned backward as much as possible to touch the upper palate.

Meditate at the Brow Point on the constant rhythm of the heart. Keep the spine completely straight. Continue for **11 minutes**. If you choose, slowly build the time each day until you can be alert while practicing it for 31 minutes.

Comments:

This meditation gives you knowledge of the past, present, and future. It directly activates the brain to integrate new areas of the brain and balances the nervous system. If your spine is straight as you master this meditation, your entire destiny and self-concept will change and expand.

Sit in **Easy Pose** or Lotus Pose and place the palms in Prayer Pose, **9 to 12 inches in front of the chest**, at the level of the heart. Inhale and swing the head from the right shoulder across the chest to the left shoulder. Complete the swing by pulling the chin in facing straight forward. Focus at the Brow Point and project this mantra silently in perfect rhythm:

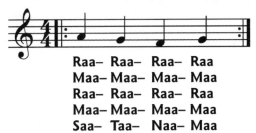

Raa– Raa– Raa– Raa
Maa– Maa– Maa– Maa
Raa– Raa– Raa– Raa
Maa– Maa– Maa– Maa
Saa– Taa– Naa– Maa

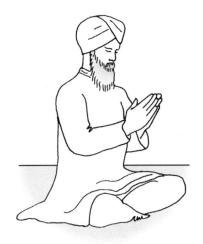

Exhale. Inhale and immediately swing the head from right to left. The head swing is quick and will give a little pull at the base of the skull. Coming to center, vibrate the mantra. Continue for **11 minutes** and with practice, gradually build up the time to 31 minutes.

Comments:

This meditation can totally reorganize the brain secretions. In Kundalini Yoga, the two halves of the brain are each divided into five main parts. These parts alternate their dominance every 2½ hours. During this kriya, the mudra and its automatic pressure on the little fingers which touch each other from the base to the tip stimulates the heart meridian and connects the first and third brain areas, correlating your desires with your actions and achievements. You become more effective.

The motion of the head puts pressure on the brain ducts to circulate the spinal fluid back into the blood stream. The circulation in the spinal fluid and meridians is often blocked at the base of the neck. This is particularly true of those who have used a drug like marijuana.

The sound of this mantra travels the mental orbit of your life. On Raa Raa Raa Raa Maa Maa Maa Maa, you travel from your central self into the orbit of mental life. "Ra" is the sun, "Ma" is the moon. You return with the *bij* mantra, "Sa Ta Na Ma." The rhythm is very important. If you cannot set the time of the mantra into a proper rhythm, the rhythm of the time cannot serve you. The moment you can reflect and create the proper rhythm of the time under the polarity of finite consciousness, then Infinity has a right to serve you.

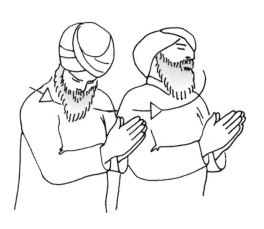

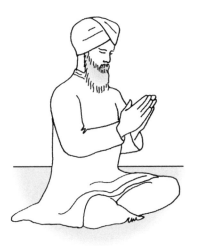

On the **fourth** and **eleventh days of the moon cycle**, there is a special pressure on the endocrine system to secrete and cleanse itself. To take advantage of this for your physical and mental health, practice this meditation for one hour on each of those days. **The kriya will have the maximum value to you on these special days**.

Guru Gobind Singh Shakti Mantra Meditation

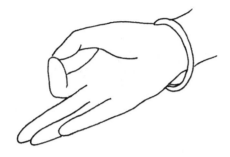

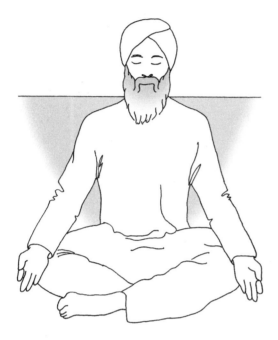

Sit in **Easy Pose** with the elbows straight and hands in **Gyan Mudra**. Close the eyes, concentrate at the Brow Point and **chant two complete cycles of this mantra with each breath.**

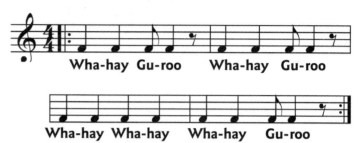

Wha-hay Gu-roo   Wha-hay Gu-roo

Wha-hay Wha-hay   Wha-hay Gu-roo

After chanting the two cycles, take a deep, quick breath and repeat. A complete cycle takes about 12 seconds. Continue for 11 to 31 minutes. Inhale and concentrate the energy at the crown of the head.

Comments:

This is the science of Laya Yoga. It is precise and exacting—and it is no one's private property. Yogi Bhajan made this available to everyone without secrecy or initiation, as was traditionally done, as a service to humanity at a time when people needed every technique available to grow and change to meet the needs of this Age.

Laya Yoga is the science of relating breath, rhythm and mantra to produce altered states of consciousness. Each *japa* (repetition of mantra) creates *tapa* (psychic heat). When you rotate the breath and volume of sound properly, it creates heat that burns off karma. Knowledge cannot be transferred properly by secret whispering in the ears of disciples; it must be an open and conscious effort by the student to expand your higher consciousness into practical expression.

A fundamental motivation and instinct in each human being is to seek happiness. Usually we search all over the world for the right time, the right place, and the right partner, but we never find them all at

one time, nor do any of them stay for long. Time, the great reaper, has its harvest of our sorrows and insecurities, but all we want is happiness. There is a state of ecstasy which exists within us all the time. It is not dependent on the caprice of circumstance and personality. It is an infinite pool that refreshes the heart and gives us strength to create a better self and a better world. It is available; we only need to access it. This meditation is the key that opens the door to that experience of ecstasy.

The mantra is a triple sound. As you continue the meditation it will lead your mind through three stages. The first stage is rhythmic and your mind will enjoy it, but it will still allow the thoughts of the day to enter. You will resist putting all your energy toward ecstasy. In the second stage, your self-conscious mind will reward you and allow you to feel yourself. However, you will feel disturbed as your usual thoughts slip away. In the third stage, you will want to get rid of the self-consciousness and immerse yourself unconsciously into the ecstasy. You will become so calm you will want to sleep. This is the merging of a raindrop into a vastly calm and beautiful lake. You reflect all, cleanse all, refresh all. If you cross this third stage, you can know the ecstasy living within yourself and enter into a conscious balance and play with the Infinity.

The relationship between your life in the finite and the Infinite depends on the rhythm of the breath. By controlling the breath, this kriya gives you a consciousness of ecstasy and calms the nerves. This calmness can also help to reduce fevers.

Sit in a comfortable pose. Straighten the spine and make sure the first six lower vertebrae are locked forward. Make fists of both hands and extend the thumbs straight. **Place the thumbs** on the temples and find the niche where the thumbs just fit. This is the lower anterior portion of the frontal bone above the temporal-sphenoid suture; just outside and slightly above the eyebrow.

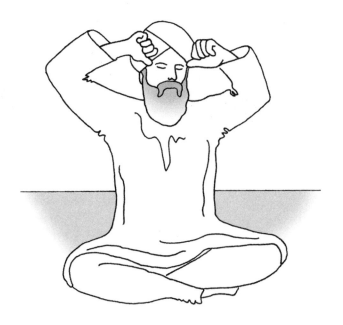

Lock the back molars together and keep the lips closed. Contract the jaw muscles, alternating the pressure on and off the molars in a steady pulsation. Your thumbs are placed correctly if you feel the muscle under the thumbs move with the pulsation. Feel it massage the thumbs and apply a firm pressure with the hands.

Keep the eyes closed and concentrate at the Brow Point. Silently vibrate the five primal sounds, **Sa Ta Na Ma**, at the brow in rhythm with the jaw's contractions. Continue **5–7 minutes**. With practice the time can be increased to 20 minutes and ultimately to 31 minutes.

Comments:

This meditation is one of a class of meditations that will become well-known and useful to future medical practice as we empower each person to participate in their own healing. Yogi Bhajan called these "Medical Meditations" because they were so effective and targeted for particular needs. Meditation will be used to alleviate all kinds of mental and physical afflictions, but it will be many years before the new medical science will understand the effects of this kind of meditation well enough to delineate all its parameters in measurable factors. While research is slow and revelatory to the mechanisms, we can use these procedures now for immediate help based on their long clinical history; they are open to everyone and not intended to be a tool only professionals can apply.

The pressure exerted by the thumbs triggers a rhythmic reflex that causes the central brain to adjust its secretions. The yogis also linked this stimulation to the activation of an area directly underneath the stem of the pineal gland which helps coordinate and control the pituitary function—a mechanism yet to be explored medically. An imbalance in this area makes mental and physical addictions seemingly unbreakable.

In modern culture, the imbalance is pandemic. If we are not addicted to smoking, eating, drinking or drugs, then we are addicted subconsciously to acceptance, advancement, rejection, emotional love, etc. All these lead us to insecure and neurotic behavior patterns.

The imbalance in this pineal area upsets the radiance of the pineal gland itself. The yogis considered the stone-like disposition of the pineal as it ages as a functional change that made it sensitive to more subtle connections to the aura. It is this pulsating subtle radiance that regulates the pituitary gland via the chakra system as well as through more direct neurotransmitter links. Because the pituitary regulates the rest of the glandular system, the entire body and mind go out of balance when the pineal pulse is off. This meditation corrects the problem. It is excellent for everyone but particularly effective for rehabilitation efforts in drug dependence, mental illness, and phobic conditions.

Wahe Guru Kriya for Nervous Balance

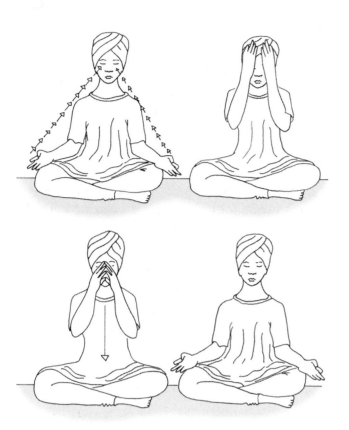

Sit in Lotus or **Easy Pose**. Rest the hands on the knees in Gyan Mudra. The eyes are almost closed—about 1/10 open. Break the **inhale into 10 equal parts** or "sniffs." As you inhale, release the mudra, turn the palms up with the fingers straight; with each segment of the inhale, move the hands in small mechanical jerks one-tenth of the way toward the forehead. On the tenth inhale, the palms come to the forehead with the base of the palms covering the eyebrows and the fingers pointing straight up. As you exhale, join the corresponding fingertips of each hand, with the palms separated. Bring the hands down the center line slowly as you exhale. Smoothly separate the hands as they reach the level of the Navel Point and return them to the original position with Gyan Mudra on the knees. On each inhale mentally vibrate the mantra, **Wahe**. On the exhale vibrate, **Guru**. Continue for **3–11 minutes**.

Comments:

This kriya builds the nervous system so that nothing bothers you. It stimulates the pituitary and gives you an expanded intuitive sense; it makes the mind clear and decisive. If the aura and nerves lack strength, it is difficult to act on your ideals. This kriya helps you direct yourself with consciousness and courage. Begin the practice with only a few minutes then build slowly up to 11 minutes.

■ Guru Ram Das Rhythmic Harmony for Happiness

Sit in a peaceful meditative pose. Keep the eyes ¹/₁₆ open. Men form Shuni Mudra with the left hand, thumb and middle finger touch; and Ravi Mudra with the right hand, thumb and ring finger touch. Women reverse the mudras. Rest the hands on the knees. Chant in a soft monotone:

Guru Guru Wahe Guru, Guru Ram Das Guru

Each repetition takes about 8 to 10 seconds. Continue for **11 to 31 minutes**.

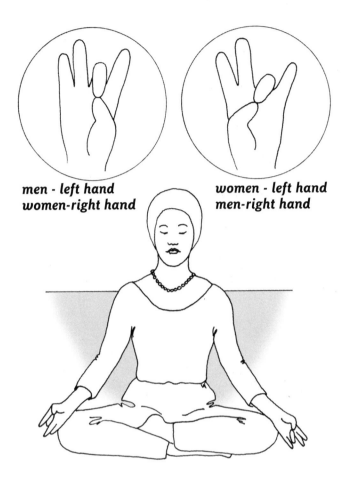

men - left hand
women-right hand

women - left hand
men-right hand

Comments:

When Yogi Bhajan taught this meditation he said: "It brings to the self a meditative peace. This is a *maithuna*. It's so vibratory even your lips, your upper palate, your tongue, your entire surroundings feel a vibratory effect. It's my personal mantra. It was given to me by Guru Ram Das in his astral self, not when I was challenged, but when Guru Ram Das was challenged. The beauty of this mantra is that it was tested. When our lives were in danger I said, 'Folks, keep on chanting this. We'll always be protected.' It's the same today. It always will be through every moment of life. It is called ecstasy of consciousness. The impossible becomes pure, simple, truthfully possible because you have the given values and you have given yourself—soul and spirit—to those given values righteously. It is then that God manifests everything. And that's why we chant in this mudra this simple mantra."

Brahm Mudra Meditation

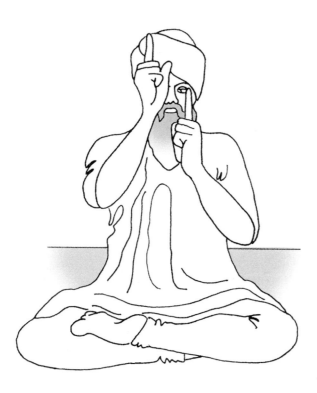

Sit with the spine straight. Make fists of both hands. The thumb should be on the outside of the fist with Jupiter fingers pointing straight up. Hold the two hands so that they face each other. The left hand is lower, the left Jupiter fingertip being exactly even with the lower knuckle of the right thumb. The two hands are like conches pointing to God. The eyes are open, looking straight and directly at, and through, the space of the hands. Hold the hands about 1½ feet from the face. Keep the neck straight. **Mentally meditate on Aad Guray Nameh, Jugaad Guray Nameh, Sat Guray Nameh, Siree Guroo Dayv-ay Nameh**. *I bow to the primal wisdom. I bow to the wisdom true through the ages. I bow to the true wisdom. I bow to the great unseen wisdom.*

After 11 minutes close the eyes and, holding the position, **chant the mantra aloud** in a monotone with a simple, moderate rhythm.

Comments:

This mudra symbolizes yin and yang pointing toward God. It is a mudra of immediate spirit and protection. All previous incarnations, the present, and the future shall be directed toward righteousness. This mudra changes the metabolism of the mind and develops a mandala called "Brahm Mandala."

Brahm Mudra is a good tool (or technique) to moderate outrageous behavior, tremendous depression, and inconsistency in character. It creates happiness on the spot where there is unhappiness.

Sit in **Easy Pose** with a straight spine. Raise the hands up near the shoulders in front of the body. The palms face forward. With the right hand, touch the thumb tip to the tip of the little finger while keeping the other fingers extended and joined. With the left hand, touch the tips of the thumb and the ring finger while keeping the other fingers extended and joined.

To begin the meditation do nothing but concentrate on the hands and keep the fingers straight. Breathe normally. When you are sure that the mudra is correct close the eyes and project a beam of light from between the eyebrows at the root of the nose.

When you are sure that the posture and the beam are correct, the third step is to rotate mentally the mantra, **Ong Kar**, at the Heart Center.

Begin timing the practice of the meditation after the entire posture, beam and mantra are set. Continue for **11 minutes**. If can work up to half an hour you will be surprised what it can do for you.

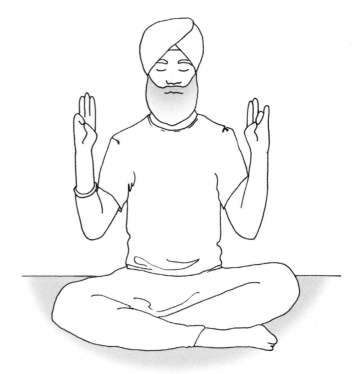

Comments:

   It is very important to stabilize the posture, the mudra, and the beam. This is a mudra practiced in China. It was brought there from Ceylon in the 14th or 15th century by a *sadhu* who was sent by his Chinese Emperor. If you ever want to talk to your mind, this is the mudra. It was used to control the mind and to have the mind follow the consciousness instead of the ego. This is the very definition of free will in yoga and is every person's right in this life. We normally do not use it. We react out of impulse or to escape pain. This meditation uses the refined capacity of the mind to rise above pain, reactions and ego to guide your actions from your own free will and consciousness.

Trikuti Turvani Kriya

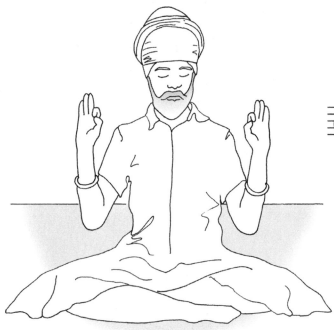

Sit in Easy Pose or other comfortable seated position with a straight spine. Bring the hands into **Gyan Mudra at shoulder height**—three or four inches wider than the shoulders—palms facing forward. This is called Dhyan Mudra.

The **eyes look at the tip of the nose**. Deeply inhale and completely exhale as the mantra is chanted **three times on one breath**.

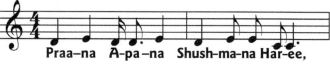

Praa–na A–pa–na Shush–ma–na Har–ee,

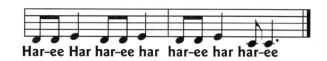

Har–ee Har har–ee har har–ee har har–ee

Be sure to chant all three repetitions of the mantra on only one breath. Chant the mantra in a fairly rapid rhythm, pronouncing each word properly. The mantra may be chanted at any pitch.

This mantra is challenging to translate directly. It describes the flow of the life force: Inflow of Cosmic Energy, outflow of Cosmic Energy, balance of Cosmic Energy through the central channel, Manifested Creativity. The three *gunas* are invoked, *'haree har, haree har, haree har'* and then manifested through the final word, *'Haree,'* your projected consciousness at the Brow Point, and the flow of the Universe within you.

Comments:

This mantra should be in every survival backpack. As we enter a period of time with high background radiation from our nuclear ambitions and from natural causes of climate and ozone changes this will be very useful. It balances your energy from the inside so you can deal with the outside.

There is no recommended time limit. Yogi Bhajan noted that "it is timeless. . . . I have to proceed with this meditation because there is so much radiation in the atmosphere that your nerves cannot stand it, and you get grouchy and upset. Those who have poor sympathetic nervous systems cannot keep their cool, and they do wrong things. . . . In the case of atomic energy radiation or total destruction, if you perfect your mind with this it may help you. . . . The simpler you make it, the happier you will be. It works fast and it is very sure. It is one of the most sacred mantras. It is so sacred I will pay your airfare, plus a thousand dollars, if you can find a single person who can repeat it to you. . . . This kriya works right on the spot.

It's not that you chant it today, it will work tomorrow. It will work right there. . . . As much as you will chant, that much it will return to you. It will cut out the karma and that much dharma will enter. It takes care of your entire texture. *Trikuti* is the triangle at the third eye, the individual. *Turvani* means cosmic triangle, where the flows meet. These two triangles are very important. . . . People who eat meat, people who kill other animals, and take in their bad vibes, and then in return complete their cycle [the animal's], this redeems them. This is actually the offering to God, and it's a most beautiful offering of *praana*. . . . This mantra can stop the cosmic disturbance. In very, very old times when typhoons used to come, when destruction used to come from heavens, people used to practice this mantra. When they thought there was no escape, they would sit down together, meditate and chant. Somehow miracle of God, hand of God, would save them. . . . This is the basic mantra."

Sarb Gyan Kriya

Sit straight in a cross-legged position. Both hands are in **Gyan Mudra in front of the Heart Center**. The palms are up and the elbows are relaxed down. Bring mudra together so that the four finger tips—thumbs and index fingers–are touching. Cross the remaining three fingers of the right hand over those of the left, keeping the fingers straight. The eyes are closed. Begin chanting **Ek Ong Kaar Sat Gur Prasaad, Sat Gur Prasaad Ek Ong Kaar**. *God and We are One. I know this by the Grace of the True Guru. I know this by the Grace of the True Guru. That God and We are One.* (Nirinjan Kaur's version is recommended.)

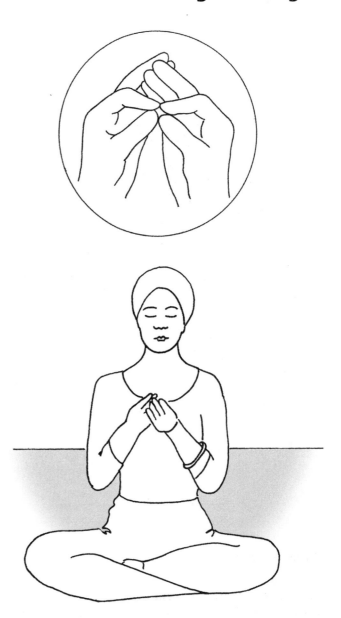

Continue for **31 minutes**. To end: inhale deeply, hold and extend the arms straight up with the palms together; the body will distribute the energy through neutral channels. Exhale. Repeat once more then inhale deeply, press the hands together and synchronize the body from toe to top. Relax.

Comments:

The name means an action that brings all knowledge and wisdom. We lose the wisdom by becoming too narrow, limited and afraid. This mantra projects the mind in a symmetrical relationship of the finite and the Infinite. Most people do not use the true depth of the mind's subtle potential. For that to open, we need to connect and project the mind from our immediate sensory spectrum into the total sense of the universe. We are a living flow of all that information and being. This simple meditation reorients the process of the mind and our sense of connection with the universe.

"As one obtains true happiness, intercommunication evolves from sexual to sensual, social, local, national, international, and cosmic to the Infinite. Out of that *prakirti*—the universe—is born. The mantra, **Ek Ong Kar Sat Gur Prasad, Sat Gur Prasad Ek Ong Kar** explains it, and this most sacred kriya is the seal to go with it. The mudra by itself will change the flow of the body's energy. Do this kriya, make it part of your life and you will be surprised at the changes in you."

161

Sanjeevanee Kriya

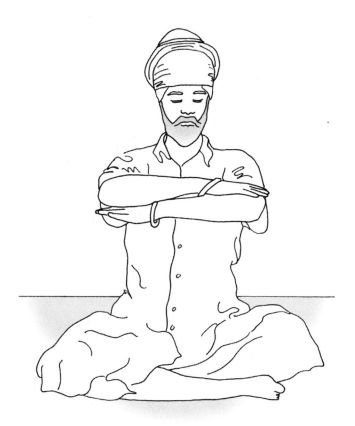

Sit in a comfortable meditative posture with a straight spine, either with the legs crossed or in a chair with the weight of both feet equally distributed on the ground.

Extend both arms straight out in front of the body parallel to the ground. Bend at the elbows and draw the forearms in toward each other until the right forearm is directly on top of the left forearm. Keep the arms parallel to the ground at all times; **don't let them drop**. The fingers are straight and pressed together; the thumbs rest in the fold of the elbows.

The eyes are $^1/_{10}$ open.

Take a breath and chant the following mantra as the breath is exhaled:

Sat Naam Sat Naam Sat Naam Sat Naam Sat Naam Sat Naam Wha-hay Guroo

Focus on the mantra. Keep the arms parallel to the ground and the spine perfectly straight at all times. Begin with **31 minutes** and build to as long as is possible.

Comments:

For stability and steadiness in your personality; this kriya empowers your word to be conscious and effective. Yogi Bhajan says it "reinvigorates the life" and "when a lot of things don't work, this never fails."

For Endless Courage and Endurance Against the Entire Universe

To be practiced at twilight.

Sit in Easy Pose. Lock your hands in **Bear Grip** at the **Heart Center**. Right palm faces inward, left palm faces outward. Eyes are at the tip of the nose.

Begin to rock the body forward about 4–6 inches, and then back to center. This is a slow, continuous, fluid movement. Move forward and back about 8 times per 10 seconds. Let the body move by itself. Do not apply physical muscle.

Chant the mantra, **Har**, each time you move forward. Chant in the following manner: Turn the tip of the tongue back so it strikes the upper pallet each time you chant. The word comes out sounding more like "Hu(d)-uh." Generate the sound of the mantra from the center of the mouth. **Har** is one of the aspects of God—the Creative Infinity. Continue for **11 minutes**.

To finish: Inhale, suspend the breath for 20 seconds, and then pull on the Bear Grip with all the power in your hands, so the energy can be displaced to every part and fiber of the body. Repeat two more times.

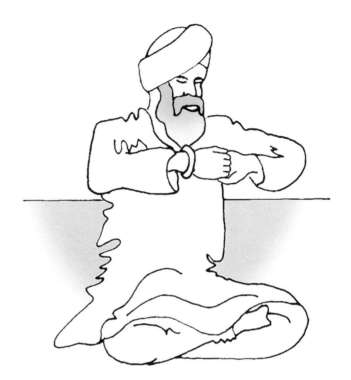

Comments:

One of the hallmarks of the yoga lifestyle is to pay attention to the rhythms of nature that we are part of. As we express our creativity in our culture, business enterprises and other activities we can easily get out of touch with the fundamentals of our biology, our patterns of energy and the cycles of the day. This meditation is done at twilight, as our energy naturally shifts. We take advantage of that shift and direct the change to give us strength.

Yogi Bhajan commented "If the tongue is properly kept turned inside the mouth, and you start chanting, *Har*, you will understand the English word 'ecstasy.' It is just a balance between the lower back, spinal cord, you, and the tongue. It can change your vibration, nervous system, and your central nerve, to be so strong that after practice you can become very fearless.

"Most things we do out of fear. We think we love, but we don't. In our life, love is our attachment to emotions, and fear is our constriction of our self-power. Both are bad. Actually, when you are really in love you are humongous. Nothing can stop you. If you are afraid, you freeze, you can't move properly.

"You have two things in life to do: Carry the day and carry the night. You want to go to work to carry the work. Wrong. You have a date at night; you want to carry the date. Wrong. You carry the day and you carry the night. God has given you two twilights, 4 to 7 in the morning and 4 to 7 in the evening."

163

Tapa Yog Karam Kriya

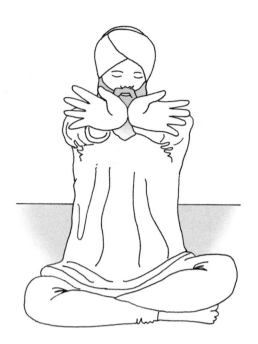

Sit in a meditative pose. Bring the palms together and extend the arms straight forward parallel to the ground. Press the wrists together and extend the hands, spread the palms and fingers as wide apart as you can, as though pushing against a wall. The eyes are slightly open looking down at the tip of the nose. Begin rhythmically chanting: **Sat Nam, Sat Nam, Sat Nam, Sat Nam, Sat Nam, Sat Nam, Wahe Guru**. Continue for **11 minutes**.

Comments:

We can improve our caliber to deliver our intentions and act effectively by developing a will that takes us past the demoting habits that interfere with our conscious efforts. When we guide ourselves and are no longer at the mercy of subconscious habits, then we become the master of the Self. But overcoming old habits and starting new ones requires strong nerves and willpower. This kriya develops willpower and gives you the capacity to understand the elements of your personality. You can know what you are thinking and regulate the flow of those thoughts. This kriya is a perfect sadhana for those who have difficulty completing projects and fulfilling intentions.

Meditation for the Lower Triangle

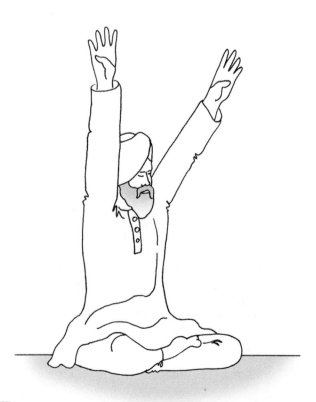

Sit in **Easy Pose**. Make sure the spine is tall and straight. Bring the thumbs of both hands onto the mound just below the little finger. Extend the right arm straight up hugging the ear. Extend the left arm to 60° from horizontal, with the wrist straight and the palm facing downward. Keep the eyes slightly open. Look down toward the upper lip. Press the elbows straight. Stretch the arms up from the shoulders. Continue for **11 minutes**.

Comments:

This meditation alleviates any problem in the lower spine. It directly heals problems related to the kidneys and adrenal glands. It helps repair the energy drained by long-term stress. It also helps the heart. Although there is no breath specified, the breath will automatically become longer and deeper as you continue. It is important to hold the arms perfectly still to receive the full benefit of this meditation.

Sit in Lotus or **Easy Pose**. Arch the arms up over the head with the palms facing down. If you are male, put the right palm on top of the left. Females put the left palm on top of the right. Bring the tips of the thumbs together, pointing back behind you. The arms are slightly bent at the elbows. Keep the eyelids open slightly and look down toward the upper lip.

Chant the mantra **Wahe Guru**. Form the sounds with the lips and tongue very precisely. **Whisper** it so that Guru is almost inaudible. It takes about 2½ seconds per repetition. Continue for **11 minutes**.

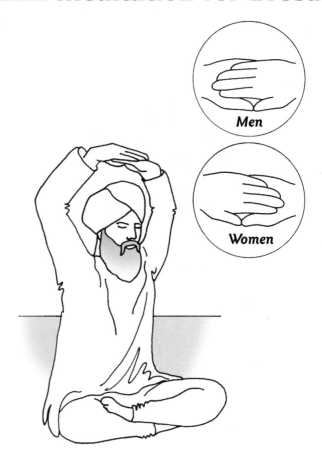

Men

Women

Comments:

This kriya is very potent and must be respected. When beginning, limit the time to a maximum of 11 minutes. Then increase the time by 1 minute every 15 days, until you reach a total of 31 minutes. The effects are extensive. The meditation affects the element of trust in the human personality. Trust is the basis of faith and commitment and the sense of reality. It will give you the elevation of spirit so you can stand up to any challenge. It builds and balances the aura from the Fourth Chakra up.

Meditation for Human Quality

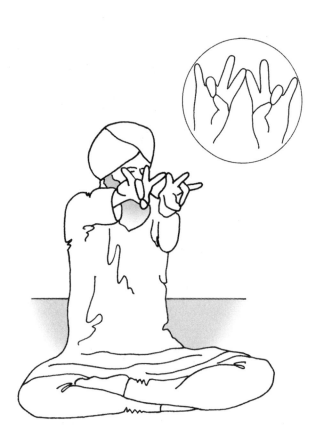

Sit in an easy cross-legged pose, keeping the spine straight. With both hands, form **Ravi Mudra**: Touch the tip of the ring finger to the tip of the thumb. Extend both arms forward with the palms down. Spread the three fingers wide and keep them straight. Bring the sides of the first joint of the index fingers together. Raise the arms slightly so that the index fingers are at the level of the eyes. **Keep the eyes relaxed and open** and the arms straight. Look over the index fingers to the horizon. Hold this position completely steady and still. Continue for **a maximum of 11 minutes**.

Comments:

As human beings we are filled with extraordinary qualities that define us, such as creativity, compassion, devotion, kindness, endurance and intention. When we feel blocked in our life, we often need to call on these and not rely on reactions and emotional reflexes. These qualities need the support of the Third, Fourth and Fifth Chakras to be strong and available to us. The First and Second Chakras are below human. The Sixth, Seventh and Eighth Chakras are beyond human. So it is only in the area of the heart that we can fulfill our nature. The Heart Center is the first chakra at which we have a distinct sense of our self. The Fifth Chakra adds the power to project and manifest that quality. This meditation opens the power of the Fourth Chakra; balances and repairs the sympathetic nervous system; helps the physical heart; and gives resistance to tension and high pressure environments. The greatest result is that it connects you with the inner sense of being human.

Sit in an Easy Pose, with a light jalandhar bandh.

Eye Position: The eyes are closed looking straight ahead at the back of the eyelids.

Mudra: Bring the elbows to rest on the ribs, forearms extended in front of you, with the hands in front of the heart, right over left, palms up. The hands are approximately 10 degrees higher than the elbows. There is no bend in the wrists. The arms from the fingertips to the elbows form a straight line. The left side of the right hand, along the mound of Mars, should lay over the Life Line of the left hand so that the Heart Line of the right hand effectively intersects the Life Line of the left hand. The thumbs are extended out to the sides of the hands, the fingertips and palms are slightly offset.

Mantra: Mentally chant the mantra:

Har har wha-hay gu-roo

Breath & Visualization: Inhale through the nostrils, pull back on the navel, and suspend the breath. Mentally chant the mantra for as long as you are able while retaining the breath. While chanting, visualize your hands surrounded by white light. Exhale through the nostrils and visualize lightning shooting out from your fingertips. When you have completely exhaled, hold the breath out, pull mulbandh, and again mentally recite the mantra as long as you are able. Inhale deeply and continue.

Recommended time of practice is 31-62 minutes.

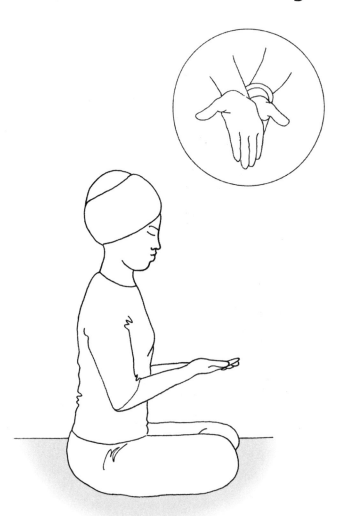

Comments:

Yogi Bhajan referred to this kriya as Tershula Kriya, the thunderbolt of Shiva, or Sidh Karm Kriya. This meditation was also taught visualizing blue light surrounding the hands. Trishula is the thunderbolt of Shiva (one of the Hindu Trinity of gods): Brahma, Vishnu and Shiva, Shiva is the destroyer or regenerator. Trishula can activate the self-healing process. This meditation balances the three gunas—the three qualities that permeate all creation: *rajas*, *tamas*, and *sattva*. It brings the three nervous systems together. It gives you the ability to heal at a distance, through your touch or through your projection. Many psychological disorders or imbalances in the personality can be cured through practice of this kriya, and it is helpful in getting rid of phobias, especially father phobia.

It is suggested that this meditation be done in a cool room, or at night when the temperature is cooler, since it directly stimulates the kundalini and generates a great deal of heat in the body.

Glossary

3HO: Healthy, Happy, Holy Organization. Begun by Yogi Bhajan in 1969 upon his teaching career in the West.

Aquarian Age: The next in a succession of astrological ages each lasting roughly 2,000 years. Fully inaugurated in 2012, the Aquarian Age will witness a radical change in consciousness, human sensitivity, and technology. The central change of this new age emphasizes an increased sensitivity and evolution of our power of awareness and a new relationship to our mind.

Amrit Vela: Literally "ambrosial time." It is the 2½ hours before the rise of the sun. During this special time you are most receptive to the soul; you can clear the subconscious of wrong habits and impulses; and you can connect with the teachers and saints from all traditions. It is the best time to perform sadhana (spiritual discipline).

Antar, Bantar, Jantar, Mantar, Tantar, Patantar, and Sotantar: These describe the sequence of creative expression from inner essence to full manifestation. Antar is the inner essence and being. It is before form. Each essence has an associated structure in time and space, a dimension to it, bantar. This structure is fulfilled by an appropriate matching set of qualities, jantar, which has a unique sound resonance, mantar, and a distinct visual form, yantar. This form and energy interrelate to the universe, tantar, creating a projection and track as it threads through time and space, patantar, until finally achieving its liberated form, beyond time and space, sotantar. This form creates a neutral point that ties together many of the polarities inherent in Prakirti to embed and express the essence of the antar in creation.

Apana: The eliminating force of the body.

Aradhana: Refers to the second stage in the steps toward mastery: sadhana, aradhana, prabhupati; discipline, attitude, and mastery, respectively. It is the conscious practice of connecting the Self to the Infinite Self.

Arcline: One of 10 bodies or containing vehicles of a human being. It is a shiny thin arc that goes from ear to ear over the forehead near the normal hairline. It reflects the interaction of the soul of the person with its vital energy resources, and in it are written the potential, destiny, and health of the person.

Ardas: Prayer, a formal prayer offered by the Sikhs

Asana: Seat or posture.

Atma: The soul or finite form of the Infinite in consciousness. It is transcendental in nature, not a product of the mind but a part of pure awareness. It is a witness of everything and can only be revealed through itself.

Aura: The radiant field of energy and consciousness that surrounds the physical body and which holds and organizes the seven centers of energy called chakras. Its strength, measured by brightness and radius, determines the vitality, mental concerns, and psychophysical integrity of a person.

Awareness: The pure nature of existence; the power to be consciously conscious without an object or need. A fundamental property of the soul and true self; it is Kundalini as it folds and unfolds itself in existence.

Bana: A specified clothing that projects a consciousness.

Bandh: Lock—applied to the body areas and direct the prana and apana. The locks are the basic techniques that accumulate the effects of the efforts of the practitioner. They establish an equilibrium in the body. The three primary locks are Neck Lock (jalandhar bandh), Diaphragm Lock (uddiyana bandh) and Root Lock (mulbandh). When practiced together they become the Great Lock (mahabandh)

Breath of Fire: Also called agni praan. It is a rapid, rhythmical breath pattern, generated from the navel point and diaphragm with an equal inhale and exhale and usually done through the nose. It is both stimulating and relaxing. It heals, strengthens the nerves, and clears out old patterns and toxins.

Chakra: The word connotes a wheel in action. It usually refers to the seven primary energy centers in the aura that align along the spine from its base to the top of the skull. Each chakra is a center of consciousness with a set of values, concerns, and powers of action associated with it.

Chitta: The mind that permeates all that exists in nature, Universal Mind. It is part of Prakirti, transcendental nature. It is not a single state of consciousness but rather the conditions and material that allow consciousness and experience through the senses. (See also: Universal Mind.)

Consciousness: The nature of the self and being. In the realm of nature, awareness becomes consciousness. It is from the being itself. Being is expressed in consciousness through contrasts and sensations, in awareness through merger, clarity, and reality.

Dharma: A path of righteous living. It is both an ideal of virtue and a path of action that is infused with clear awareness and comprised of actions that are the soul in total synchrony with the universe. It is action without reaction or karma.

Functional Minds: The three minds (Negative, Positive, and Neutral) that act as guides for the personal sense of self.

Golden Chain or Golden Link: Historically it is the long line of spiritual masters who have preceded us. Practically it is the subtle link between the consciousness of a student and the master, which has the power to guide and protect the energy of a teaching and its techniques. This link requires the student to put aside the ego and limitations and act in complete synchrony or devotion to the highest consciousness of the master and teachings.

Gunas: The three qualities or threads that make up the fundamental forces in nature and the mind. Their interactions give motion to the world, stir the larger Greater Mind, and make up the realm of our experience. They are considered inseparable and occur in un-limited combinations. They are abstract; you can only see their effects. They are the sattva guna for clarity and purity; the rajasic guna for action and transformation, and the tamasic guna for heaviness, solidity, and ignorance.

Guru: That which takes us from ignorance to knowledge; from darkness, gu, to light, ru. It can be a person, a teaching, or in its most subtle form—the Word.

Gyan Mudra: A common hand position used in exercise and meditation, is formed by touching the tip of the index finger to the tip of the thumb. Its effect is receptivity, balance, and gentle expansion.

Humanology: A complete system of psychology to promote human excellence and spirit. It incorporates the technology of Kundalini Yoga and meditation, the use of the Shabd Guru, and the principles of spiritual counseling.

Ida: One of the three major channels (nadis) for subtle energy in the body. It is associated with the flow of breath through the left nostril and represents the qualities of the moon—calmness, receptivity, coolness, and imagination. It is associated with the functions of the parasympathetic nervous system but is not identical to it nor derived from it.

Japji Sahib: A mantra, poem, and inspired religious scripture composed by Guru Nanak. Japji Sahib gives a view of the cosmos, the soul, the mind, the challenge of life, and the impact of our actions. Its 40 stanzas are a source of many mantras and can

be used as a whole or in part to guide both your mind and your heart.

Japa: Literally "to repeat." It is the conscious, alert, and precise repetition of a mantra.

Karma: The law of cause and effect applied to mental, moral, and physical actions. Ego attaches us to and identifies us with objects, feelings, and thoughts. These attachments create a bias toward certain lines of action. Instead of acting you begin reacting. Karmas are the conditions required in order to balance or complete these tendencies. Though necessary, karma is not dictatorial or fatalistic. It is the mechanism that allows the finite experience of existence to maintain and stabilize itself. We all have free will and can take actions to re-direct the momentum of a karma. We can transform it or neutralize it using meditation, jappa, good deeds, or intuition that remove your sense of ego and the identification with that past line of action.

Kirtan: Traditional singing. Call and response or harmonizing.
Kriya: Literal meaning is "completed action." A Kundalini Yoga Kriya is a sequence of postures and yoga techniques used to produce a particular impact on the psyche, body, or self. The structure of each kriya has been designed to generate, organize, and deliver a particular state or change of state, thereby completing a cycle of effect. These effects have been codified and elaborated by Yogi Bhajan and form the basic tools used in yoga and its therapeutic applications.

Kundalini Yoga: It is a Raaj Yoga that creates vitality in the body, balance in the mind, and openness to the spirit. It is used by the householder, busy in the world, to create immediate clarity. The fourth Guru in the Sikh tradition, Guru Ram Das, was acknowledged as the greatest Raaj Yogi. (See Raaj Yogi.) He opened this long secret tradition to all.

Laya: Merging the finite with the Infinite through sound, mantra, and rhythm, and a sensitivity to its subtle structure. Often practiced in groups.

Mahan Tantric: A Master of White Tantric Yoga. This title and function was bestowed upon Yogi Bhajan in 1971. There is only one Mahan Tantric alive on the earth at any one time.

Mantra: Sounds or words that tune or control the mind. Man means mind. Tra-ng is the wave or movement of the mind. Mantra is a wave, a repetition of sound and rhythm that directs or controls the mind. When you recite a mantra you have impact: through the meridian points in the mouth, through its meaning, through its pattern of energy, through its rhythm, and through its naad—

energetic shape in time. Recited correctly a mantra will activate areas of the nervous system and brain and allow you to shift your state and the perceptual vision or energetic ability associated with it.

Maya: The creative power of the Creator that restricts and limits. It creates the sense of limitation that leads us to identify with experience, the ego, and things. Because of this it is often thought of as the illusion that blocks us from the spirit. But, as Guru Nanak (see Sikh Gurus) reminds us, you need not be attached to the productions of maya. Instead they can be used to serve and express the higher consciousness and spirit. Maya is simply Karta Purkh, the doing of the Great Being. Maya takes the ineffable into the realm of the measurable.

Meditation: Dhyan. It is a process of deep concentration or merger into an object or a state of consciousness. Meditation releases reactions and unconscious habits and build the spontaneous and intuitive link to awareness itself.

Mudra: Mudra means "seal." It usually refers to hand positions used in meditation and exercise practices. These hand positions are used to seal the body's energy flow in a particular pattern. More generally it can refer to other locks, bandhas (see mulbandh), and meditation practices that seal the flow of energy by concentration.

Mulbandh: This literally means "root lock." It is a body lock used to balance prana and apana (see prana) at the navel point. This releases reserve energy which is used to arouse the Kundalini. It is a contraction of the lower pelvis—the navel point, the sex organs, and the rectum.

Naad: The inner sound that is subtle and all-present. It is the direct expression of the Absolute. Meditated upon, it leads into a sound current that pulls the consciousness into expansion.

Naam (Nam): The manifested identity of the essence. The word derives from Naa-ay-ma, which means "that which is not, now is born." A Naam gives identity, form, and expression to that which was only essence or subtle before. It is also referred to as the Word.

Naam Simran: This refers to the state and act of deep meditation by dwelling and merging into the names of the Infinite, of God.

Nadi: Channels or pathways of subtle energy. It is said that there are over 72,000 primary ones throughout the body.

Navel Point: The sensitive area of the body near the umbilicus that accumulates and stores life force. It is the reserve energy from this area that initiates the flow of the Kundalini energy from the base of the spine. If the navel area is strong, your vital force and health are also strong.

Negative Mind: One of the three Functional Minds. It is the fastest and acts to defend you. It asks, "How can this harm me? How can this limit or stop me?" It is also the power to just say no, stop something, or reject a direction of action.

Neutral Mind: The most refined and often the least developed of the three Functional Minds. It judges and assesses. It witnesses and gives you clarity. It holds the power of intuition and the ability to see your purpose and destiny. It is the gateway for awareness.

Pavan Guru: Literally, the "breath of the guru." It is the transformative wisdom that is embedded in the patterns of breath, especially those patterns generated in the expression of naad in sound or mantra.

Pingala: One of the three major channels (nadis) for subtle energy in the body. It is associated with the flow of breath through the right nostril and represented the qualities of the sun—energy, heat, action, and projective power. It is associated with the functions of the sympathetic nervous system but is not identical to it or derived from it.

Positive Mind: One of the three Functional Minds. It elaborates, magnifies, extends, and assists. It asks, "How can this help me? How can I use this? What is the positive side of this?"

Prabhupati: Literally means "spouse of God". This is the state of mastery in the practitioner. A state of neutrality is reached and prabhupati represents the opening and atunement to the superconscious.

Prakirti: Transcendental Nature. It is creation as we can experience it. It includes mind and matter. It is formed from the motion and interaction of the gunas. It is multi-leveled and evolved from the original consciousness of the Absolute.

Prana: The universal life force that gives motion. It is the breath in air. It is the subtle breath of the purusha as it vibrates with a psychophysical energy or presence. Prana regulates the modes and moods of the mind.

Pranayam: Regulated breathing patterns or exercises.

Pratyahaar: One of the eight limbs of yoga, it is the synchronization of the thoughts with the Infinite. To quote Yogi Bhajan; "Pratyahaar is the control of the mind through withdrawal of the senses. The joy in your life, which you really want to enjoy, is within you. There is nothing more precise than you within you. The day you find the you within you, your mind will be yours. In pratyahaar we bring everything to zero (shuniaa), as pranayam brings everything to Infinity."

Projection: A stance of the psyche projecting into action. It is an attitude of your mind that is a tendency to approach action in a certain way. There are 27 Projections that arise from the nine Aspects of the mind interacting with the three Functional Minds. Purkha: The great Being of existence.

Purusha: The transcendental self, soul, atma, or spirit. It is the first contained embodiment of the unlimited consciousness and is formed with the subtle body. It is the consciousness and witness of the spirit that indwells the body.

Raaj Yogi: A yogi who follows the royal or highest path. One who excels and exalts the self in the midst of life without monastic withdrawal. One who places the self on the throne and presides with consciousness over all domains of manifestation, internal and external. (See Kundalini Yoga, Yogi.)

Sadhana: A spiritual discipline; the early morning practice of yoga, meditation, and other spiritual exercises.

Saa-Taa-Naa-Maa: This is referred to as the Punj Shabd Mantra (panj means five). It is the "atomic" or naad form of the mantra Sat Naam. It is used to increase intuition, balance the hemispheres of the brain, and to create a destiny for someone when there was none.

Sadhu: A traditional term for a Yogi, one who leads the life of an ascetic, removed from the world.

Sat: Existence; what is; the subtle essence of Infinity itself, often translated as Truth.

Sat Naam: The essence or seed embodied in form; the identity of truth. When used as a greeting it means "I greet and salute that reality and truth which is your soul." It is called the Bij Mantra— the seed for all that comes.

Sattvic: One of the three basic qualities of nature (gunas). It represents purity, clarity, and light.

Shabd: Sound, especially subtle sound or sound imbued with consciousness. It is a property or emanation of consciousness itself. If you meditate on shabd it awakens your awareness.

Shabd Guru: These are sounds spoken by the Gurus; the vibration of the Infinite Being which transforms your consciousness; the sounds and words captured by the Gurus in the writings which comprise the Siri Guru Granth Sahib.

Shakti: The creative power and principle of existence itself. Without it nothing can manifest or bloom. It is feminine in nature.

Shuniya: A state of the mind and consciousness where the ego is brought to zero or complete stillness. There a power exists. It is the fundamental power of a Kundalini Yoga teacher. When you become shuniaa then the One will carry you. You do not grasp or act. With folded hands you "are not." It is then that Nature acts for you.

Shushmana: One of the three major channels (nadis) for subtle energy in the body. It is associated with the central channel of the spine and is the place of neutrality through which the Kundalini travels when awakened. When mantra is vibrated from this place it has the power of soul and consciousness.

Sikh Gurus: In the Sikh tradition there were 10 living Gurus and one Guru, the Shabd Guru—the Word that guided and flowed through each of them. This succession of 10 Gurus revealed the Sikh path over a 200-year period. They were:

1st Sikh Guru: Guru Nanak	6th Sikh Guru: Guru Hargobind
2nd Sikh Guru: Guru Angad	7th Sikh Guru: Guru Har Rai
3rd Sikh Guru: Guru Amar Das	8th Sikh Guru: Guru Har Krishan
4th Sikh Guru: Guru Ram Das	9th Sikh Guru: Guru Teg Bahadur
5th Sikh Guru: Guru Arjan	10th Sikh Guru: Guru Gobind Singh

The 10th Sikh Guru, Guru Gobind Singh, passed the Guruship to the Siri Guru Granth Sahib, which embodies the writings, teachings, and sound current of the Gurus.

Simran: A deep meditative process in which the naam of the Infinite is remembered and dwelled in without conscious effort.

Siri Guru Granth Sahib: Sacred compilation of the words of the Sikh Gurus as well as of Hindu, Muslim, Sufi, and other saints. It captures the expression of consciousness and truth derived when in a state of divine union with God. It is written in naad and embodies the transformative power and structure of consciousness in its most spiritual and powerful clarity. It is a source of many mantras.

Sunni-ae: Listening or hearing. Attuning yourself to the subtle sound current that is the unstruck sound, or Infinity.

Tamas: One of the three basic qualities of nature (gunas). It represents heaviness, slowness, and dullness. It is inertia and confusion.

Tapas: Fire or purification. Traditionally one of the qualities in the niyamas, or code of the practitioner.

Tattvas: A category of cosmic existence; a stage of reality or being; a "thatness" of differentiated qualities. In total there are 36 tattvas. Each wave of differentiation has its own rules and structure. The final five tattvas are called the gross elements and have the phasic qualities and relationships of ether, air, fire, water, and earth.

Ten Bodies: We are all spiritual beings having a human experience. In order to have this experience the spirit takes on 10 bodies or vehicles. They are the Soul Body, the three Mental Bodies (Negative, Positive, and Neutral Minds), the Physical Body, Pranic Body, Arcline Body, Auric Body, Subtle Body, and Radiant Body. Each body has its own quality, function, and realm of action.

Third Eye Point or Brow Point: The sixth chakra or center of consciousness. It is located at a point on the forehead between the eyebrows. Associated with the functioning of the pituitary gland, it is the command center and integrates the parts of the personality. It gives you insight, intuition, and the understanding of meanings and impacts beyond the surface of things. For this reason it is the focal point in many meditations.

Universal Mind: This refers to the entire spectrum of mental existence and sentient potential in the universe in whatever form. Mind and matter are considered gradations of transcendental nature, Prakirti, and can exist without or before a particular entity to experience it. (See also chitta.)

Vayus: The different frequencies and modes of motion of the Prana. Each vayu has a natural home in the body. They are prana, apana, udana, samana, and vyana.

Wahe Guru: A mantra of ecstasy and dwelling in God. It is the Infinite teacher of the soul. Also called the gur mantra.

Yogi: One who has attained a state of yoga (union) where polarities are mastered and transcended. One who practices the disciplines of yoga and has attained self-mastery.

Resources

This and other KRI products are available from the
Kundalini Research Institute (KRI):

www.kriteachings.org

Remember to always buy from 'The Source'!

For information regarding international events:

www.3HO.org

To find a teacher in your area:

www.ikyta.org

To become a Kundalini Yoga teacher:

www.kriteachings.org

Of further interest:

www.sikhnet.org

Kundalini Yoga as taught by Yogi Bhajan®

Kundalini Research Institute